The Insulin Resistance Diet Plan & Cookbook:

101 Vegan Recipes for Permanent Weight Loss, to Manage PCOS, Prevent Prediabetes & Metabolic Syndrome

by Patricia Karnowski MSOM

Copyright © 2016 Patricia Karnowski

ISBN: 1534813160
ISBN-13: 9781534813168

DEDICATION

I am dedicating this book to my mother, Theresa Mary Russell. It is her birthday today. She was born on June 18, 1936 and passed away on September 23, 2010. She had lived most of her adult life with diabetes and struggled with morbid obesity. She had been told that she would need to start kidney dialysis just a few weeks before she died. Oh how I wish my mother had found this healthy way of eating. I am positive she would have loved the food. She would probably still be alive to know and love all of her great grand children. I love you, Mom and I miss you.

CONTENTS

ACKNOWLEDGMENTS

I want to acknowledge authors of The China Study, Dr. T. Colin Campbell, Jacob Gould Schurman Professor Emeritus of Nutritional Biochemistry at Cornell University, and his son Thomas M. Campbell II, a physician. This book opened up a whole new way of seeing the world.

1. INTRODUCTION

Thank you for buying this diet plan & cookbook. I hope it is just what you have been looking for.

You will find the basic diet plan and 101 recipes chosen to perfectly support your goal of permanent weight loss and to prevent diabetes and metabolic syndrome which is exactly how women are able to manage polycystic ovarian syndrome (PCOS).

I have been a Practitioner of Traditional Chinese Medicine for 16 years. I specializing in helping men and women with infertility problems. This is how I ran into so many people dealing with problems related to insulin resistance.

I also have very personal reasons that me down this path of discovery. Both of my parents had type 2 diabetes (that have passed away now), a brother and sister are insulin resistant and I have PCOS that lead to ovarian cancer.
We been overweight for most of our lives. I wonder if you have tried as many diets as we have in all of these years.

I ended the dieting merry-go-round about 4 years ago. I landed on this new way of eating and it changed my approach to food and everything changed. I was shocked by the change in my body and my ability to keep my weight off.

I lost about 70 pounds eating foods that I love. This is no longer a diet. Diets come and go. This new way of eating will last a lifetime. I am not kidding about this. I LOVE the food. I switched my diet for obvious health reasons, but I continue eating this way because I LOVE THE TASTE OF THE FOOD. I actually feel deprived if I don't get it.

My patients feel the same way. Sometimes they call or email just to tell me how much they like something they just ate.

This never happened on the Atkin's Diet, the Paleo Diet, Nutrisystems, Weight Watchers, the South Beach Diet, Stillman Diet, the 500 Calorie HCG Diet, the Beverly Hills Diet, the Subway Diet or the Watermelon Diet. I never felt this way at Food Addicts in Recovery or Over Eaters Anonymous. I never felt so good even after detoxing with the Master Cleanse or juice fasting. I went gluten-free and Ketogenic and it wasn't like this. It also never happened on the Alkaline Diet or the Blood Type Diet (I am an O type), or Fit for Life, or Jenny Craig, or even the Sugar Buster's Diet. I have tried them all. This is so different.

I will explain the rules for the diet plan in the next chapter. It is going to be radical by most people's standards but so are the results. There will be a big learning curve when it comes to understanding this new lifestyle change, but you have these recipes to get you started and as a bonus I am giving you immediate access to the collection of informational videos at PCOSworld.com which I give to my patients to help them understand why this way of eating works so well.

Guess what? You get to eat heaps and piles of rice and potatoes and desserts every day if you feel like it. This is not a "no carb" diet. You will be full when you finish a meal as this is also not a deprivation diet.

I am proof of the success of this lifestyle. I am 61 years old. I am completely healthy (I had better "knock on wood"after making that statement). I take absolutely no medications. All of my blood levels for everything are completely normal, besides the fact that I have finally found a way to drop weight and keep it off in a way I never could before.

This is a diet plan and a recipe book, so I am not going to tell you all the science behind why this way of eating is so successful but I have included instant access to a bonus supplemental informational video series at no additional cost. You will find this in the Resources Chapter.

Enjoy the recipes and your journey to health, happiness, and a long life.

Warm Regards,
Patricia Karnowski MSOM, LAc

♥

2. RULES FOR THE GAME CHANGING DIET

Here are all the rules for your new way of eating. You should try as many of these foods as possible so you can find the foods you like in the combinations that you enjoy.

1. Eat 8 ounces of beans and/or legumes every single day.

They are high in protein and fiber and they have what is called a "2 meal effect". This means they will help to keep your blood sugar levels regulated for two meals. I have included many recipes to help you find interesting, delicious ways to eat them.

Hint: If you experience a lot of intestinal gas that so many people complain about when they start eating beans try adding a 2 inch strip of dried kombu seaweed to the beans while they are cooking.

Lentils
Split Peas
Great Northern Beans
White Beans
Broad (Fava) Beans
Cranberry (Roman) Beans
Kidney Beans
Lima Beans
Black Beans (Frijoles Negros)
Mung Beans
Cow peas (Black Eyed Peas)
Yellow Beans (Yellow Lentils)
Small White Beans
Pinto Beans
Black Turtle Beans
Pink Beans
Navy Beans
Adzuki Beans
Pigeon Peas (Red Gram)
Chickpeas (Garbanzo Beans, Bengal Gram)

2. Eat at least 2 to 4 cups of greens every single day.
You must eat at least 2 cups of greens every single day. It is so important that I said it twice.

Broccoli Raab
Kale
Artichokes
Spinach
Collard Greens
Parsley
Mustard Greens
Broccoli
Beet Greens

Arugula
Brussels Sprouts
Asparagus
Watercress
Bok Choy (Chinese Cabbage)
Cabbage
Romaine Lettuce (head of lettuce has no nutritional value)

3. Eat 100% Whole Grains

Hint: Be sure to read the label. If the first ingredient is whole wheat and the second ingredient is durham wheat (not a whole grain) or just "wheat" then this product will not be good for you. All the grains in the product must be WHOLE.

Whole Wheat (if you can tolerate it)
Old Fashioned Rolled Oats (Irish Oatmeal is good too)
Brown Rice
Japanese Soba Noodles
Spelt
Kamut (Khorasan)
Quinoa
Amaranth
Whole Wheat Pasta
Corn Pasta
Wild Rice
Semolina
Buckwheat Groats
Whole Grain Couscous
Rye Grain
Corn Grain (Yellow & White)
Millet
Barley
Brown Rice Noodles

4. Eat root vegetables.

These starchy foods are very satisfying. We like them and feel deprived without them. You can and should fill 1/2 of your plate with grains and root vegetables.

Sweet potatoes
Beets
Yams
Potatoes of call colors
Turnips
Jicama
Rutabaga
Cassava
Daikon

5. Eat fruits and vegetables. Most dieters try to eat only fruits and vegetables and try to stay away from grains and starches. That will not work. You will not feel satisfied and you will go back to eating the high fat and processed foods.

6. Eat but limit the quantity of the following

avocado - not more than 2 a week

nuts and seeds - not more than 2 ounces a day. A lot of these recipes call for a small amount of nuts which is how you want to eat them. Don't sit down and eat a bag of nuts, as this will slow your weight loss down.

olives - not more than about 5 in a day. (Rinse them off before eating to clean off the salt.)

dried fruits - The less you eat the faster you lose.

7. Eat all different flavors of vinegar and spices and herbs

8. Take Vitamin B12 - only 2-4 mcg. per day are needed for adults. Animal products are the main sources of B12 for most people and you will not be eating these. Vitamin B12 is made by bacteria that the animals eat. We clean our foods so well that we remove all the bacteria that produce vitamin B12 so you need to take a supplement.

9. Do not count calories - This is not a calorie restricting diet. Eat when you are hungry and eat until you are full. Portion control happens without you having to worry about it when you are eating a whole foods, plant based diet, and limiting the amount of calorie dense foods such as nuts and avocados.

DO NOT EAT THE FOLLOWING FOODS

1. No Animal Products

BEEF
PORK
CHICKEN
FISH
TURKEY
GOAT
LAMB
MILK
ICE CREAM
YOGURT
CHEESE
CREAM CHEESE
SOUR CREAM
EGGS

2. No Oil

You will be getting your oil from eating nuts and seeds. This list is not an exhaustive list of oils but only the most common ones. Anywhere you used oil to cook with in the past will be substituted with vegetable broth or any other liquid you would like to use.

Coconut oil - high in saturated fat
Corn oil
Cottonseed oil
Olive oil
Palm oil
Peanut oil
Safflower oil
Sesame oil
Soybean oil
Avocado oil
All nut oils

4. No Soy Products.

These "fake" foods are not whole foods also women with PCOS will not benefit and may even be harmed by the estrogen contained in soy.

Meat Alternatives
Miso
Soy Cheese
Soy Flour
Soy Milk
Soy Oil
Soy Nut Butter
Tofu (once in awhile it is okay to have tofu)
Whole Soybeans
Soy Yogurt

5. No Sugar or Sugar Substitutes - A little Stevia is okay

Sugar
Brown Sugar
Molasses
Honey
Agave
Coconut or palm sugar
Artificial sugar substitutes
Aspartame
Sucralose
Saccharin

6. Low Salt - You can add salt to your food at the table before you eat, but do not cook with it.

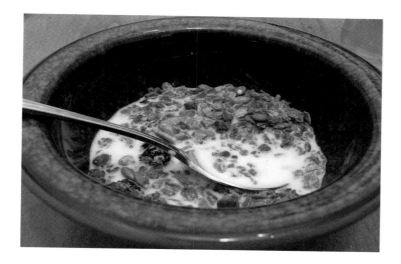

3. SUGAR FREE SWEET GRANOLA

Make your own granola rather than buying it from the store. This way you will know there is no salt, oil or sugar and the grains are 100% whole grains. Check the ingredients on the label of a box of granola. You will be shocked.

INGREDIENTS

- ½ cup water
- 6 medjool or 12 deglet dates pitted and cut into quarters
- 1½ teaspoons vanilla
- 1¼ teaspoons cinnamon
- ½ teaspoon nutmeg
- 2 cups old fashioned rolled oats
- ½ cup raisins
- ½ cup sliced almonds (optional. You will lose weight faster if you don't eat nuts.)

INSTRUCTIONS

1- Place the water, dates, vanilla, cinnamon, and nutmeg into a blender for 15 minutes.
2- Preheat oven to 250°F.
3- Line a large cookie sheet with parchment paper or use a silicone mat. You can also use a Teflon cookie sheet if there are no scratches (scratched Teflon pans are not safe).
4- Combine the rolled oats, raisins, and nuts.
5- Blend the dates, water, vanilla, cinnamon, and nutmeg until smooth.
6- Pour into the bowl of oats, raisins, and nuts, and mix with a fork.
7- Spread the granola evenly on the cookie sheet.
8- Cook on the center rack for 30 minutes.
9- Remove the pan from the oven and mix around a little.
10- Return to the oven for an additional 25 to 30 minutes.

Eat your granola with unsweetened almond milk or rice milk (women with PCOS must avoid soy milk). Store in an airtight container in the refrigerator to preserve freshness.

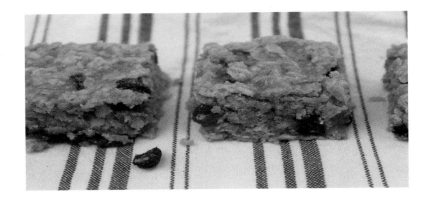

4. GRAB & GO BAKED OATMEAL APPLE RAISIN BARS

A lot of people have a hard time eating breakfast. They don't seem to be hungry in the morning. Try making a big batch of these breakfast bars. You can grab them on the way out the door in the morning and eat them on the go.

INGREDIENTS

- 2 1/2 cups old fashioned rolled oats
- 1 3/4 cups unsweetened almond or rice milk
- 1 large apple, cored, skin on, and chopped into thin pieces
- 1/2 cup raisins
- 1 1/2 teaspoons cinnamon
- 1/2 teaspoon nutmeg

INSTRUCTIONS

1. Preheat oven to 375 degrees.

2. Mix all ingredients together.

3. Spread into an 8×8-inch square Teflon (only if no scratches) baking pan lined with parchment paper or a silicone pan.

4. Bake uncovered for 30 minutes

5. Cut into snack bars

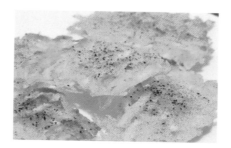

5. BETTER THAN YOUR MOM'S HASH BROWNS WITH KETCHUP

Start learning how to cook without oil. You will be shocked how easy it is.

When you made hash browns in the past you thought you had to use oil but you don't. This recipe will be a real eye-opener for you.

It is hard to eat hash browns without ketchup, but have you ever checked out the list of ingredients on the ketchup bottle in your refrigerator? Processed ketchup is filled with sugar, salt, and a lot of chemicals.

Make a big batch of ketchup so you can use it on your burgers later in the week.

INGREDIENTS

1 white or Yukon potato per person (skins on or off)
1 granulated onion, garlic and/or dried herbs of your choice to taste (I like "Mrs. Dash No Salt Table Blend")
Salt-free Ketchup (see recipe below)

INSTRUCTIONS

1. Use a food processor or the large holes of a cheese grater to grate the potatoes.

2. Preheat a non-stick skillet to medium-low heat and add the grated potatoes.

3. Cover and cook for 5 to 7 minutes.

4. When it's a medium brown color, flip the hash browns and cook for 5 to 7 more minutes.

5. Sprinkle the granulated onion and/or garlic and dried herbs on the top for the last 2 min.

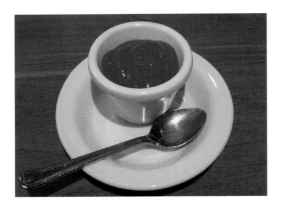

KETCHUP

INGREDIENTS

- 1 6-oz. can no-salt-added tomato paste
- 1 half of an apple diced (with or without skin)
- 1/3 cup water
- 1 tablespoon lemon juice
- ¼ teaspoon garlic powder
- ¼ teaspoon dried oregano
- 3 to 4 potatoes (wash but don't peel) cut into ¼ inch x ¼ inch lengths

INSTRUCTIONS

Combine all ingredients in a blender, food processor, Magic Bullet or Vitamix until smooth.

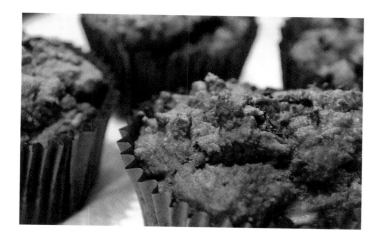

6. BLUER THAN BLUEBERRY MUFFINS

Are you shocked that you can have blueberry muffins and still lose weight? I was. The reason this recipe works is because the muffins are made with 100% whole grains and no animal fats or sugar.

The Medjool dates are a whole food. They sweeten and moisten the muffins.

To drop weight faster, only have these muffins once a week. All dried fruits are calorie dense which means they are higher in calories than fresh fruits.

INGREDIENTS

- 12 Medjool dates, pitted and chopped
- 1 cup unsweetened almond or rice milk
- 1-½ cups old fashioned rolled oats
- ¾ cup millet
- 2 teaspoons baking powder
- ½ teaspoon ground cardamom
- ½ cup unsweetened (read the label) applesauce
- 1 teaspoon lemon zest, packed
- 1 cup fresh or frozen blueberries (do not thaw first)
- ½ cup roughly chopped walnuts (Optional. You will lose weight faster without nuts.)

INSTUCTIONS

1. Preheat oven to 350 degrees.

2. Chop dates and soak them in unsweetened almond or rice milk for 15 minutes.

3. Grind oats and millet into a flour in a blender on high speed until fine and put into a mixing bowl.

4. Add the baking powder and cardamom and stir with a fork.

5. Place the dates and non-dairy milk into a blender and blend until smooth.

6. Add the date mixture to the bowl of dry ingredients along with the applesauce and lemon zest, and mix with a spoon until all the dry ingredients have disappeared.

7. Fold in the blueberries and chopped walnuts into the mixture.

8. Spoon the batter into a silicone or unscratched muffin pan filling each muffin cup about 3/4 full.

9. Bake for 30 minutes.

10. Cool in the pan for at least 15 to 20 minutes before removing.

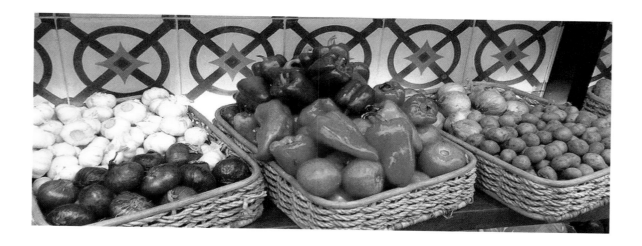

7. BREAKFAST OR ANYTIME POTATO BAKE

This recipe has a Mexican flavor. It is very rich and satisfying. The nutritional yeast has a nutty, sort-of Parmesan cheese flavor.

You must eat greens every day. Try putting them in everything you make. The smaller you cut the leaves the less you notice them and yet your body will feel so much better.

Beans are higher in protein by weight than meat, chicken, or fish.

This is actually a high fiber, high protein meal.

INGREDIENTS

- water for steaming
- 3 large russet potatoes, shredded (peeled or unpeeled)
- 2 tablespoons nutritional yeast
- water for sauteing
- ½ of a yellow onion, small diced
- 1 red or orange bell pepper, small diced
- 1 zucchini, small diced
- 8-10 sliced white mushrooms
- ½ to 1 bunch greens (kale, chard, collards, spinach, etc.) chopped into small pieces
- juice from 1 lime
- 1 tablespoon nutritional yeast
- 2 teaspoons dried basil
- 1 ½ teaspoons garlic powder
- 1 ½ teaspoons oregano
- 1 teaspoon chili powder

- ¼-½ teaspoon red pepper flakes
- 1 can diced tomatoes (no or low salt) (15-oz.)
- 1 can black beans (no salt or rinse before using) (15-oz.)
- 1 can pinto beans (no salt or rinse before using) (15-oz.)
- ½ cup chopped fresh cilantro leaves

DIRECTIONS

1. In a large pot, steam the grated potatoes (in a steamer basket) for 5-10 minutes on med-high heat until soft.

2. Separate potatoes into a two bowls. In one of the bowls, add 2 tablespoons of nutritional yeast and mix thoroughly. Set bowls aside.

3. Saute the onion, bell pepper, zucchini and mushrooms in a couple tablespoons of water for 5 minutes (adding water as needed so as not to stick); add in the greens and cook another few minutes until soft.

4. Then mix in: lime juice, dried herbs and spices, 1 tablespoon of nutritional yeast, and the steamed potatoes without the nutritional yeast.

5. Remove from heat. Fold in the remaining ingredients: tomatoes, beans and cilantro.

6. Spoon mixture into a 13×9-inch glass ungreased baking dish. Spread the remaining potato-nutritional yeast mixture on top.

7. Bake at 375 degrees for 35-45 minutes uncovered until top is lightly browned around the edges.

8. Let sit for at least 5 minutes.

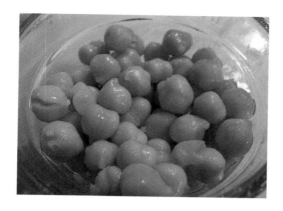

8. GARBANZO BEAN EGG-LESS OMELET

Chickpea/ garbanzo bean flour is popular in Middle Eastern and Indian cooking. It is usually found in the organic section of the grocery store in the US or a Middle Eastern market. It is a great whole grain flour to know about as it can be hard for many women with PCOS to tolerate wheat. Chickpea flour is a great alternative.

Don't expect this to taste like eggs. It has its own very nice flavor.

INGREDIENTS

- 1 cup chickpea flour
- ½ teaspoon onion powder
- ½ teaspoon garlic powder
- ¼ teaspoon white pepper
- ¼ teaspoon black pepper
- 1/3 cup nutritional yeast
- ½ teaspoon baking soda
- 3 green onions (white and green parts), chopped
- 4 ounces sauteed mushrooms (optional)

INSTRUCTIONS

1. Combine the chickpea flour, onion powder, garlic powder, white pepper, black pepper, nutritional yeast, and baking soda in a small bowl. Add 1 cup water and stir until smooth.

2. Heat a frying pan over medium heat. Pour the batter into the pan like pancakes. Sprinkle 1 to 2 tablespoons of the green onions and mushrooms onto the batter for each omelet as it cooks. Flip the omelet a couple times until both sides are brown.

3. Serve with tomatoes, spinach, salsa, hot sauce, or Sriracha sauce.

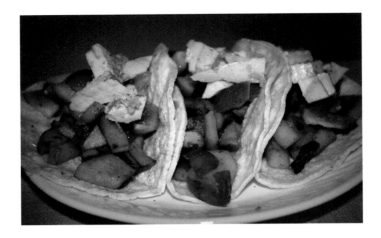

9. SIMPLE BREAKFAST TACO

Why didn't we think of sweet potatoes on tacos before? I always felt guilty eating sweet potatoes because I was afraid that they were going to make me fat. Little did I know, the real problem with sweet potatoes was the butter, sour cream, and marshmallow we put on them.

Women with PCOS can eat sweet potatoes like this every day if they want to and still lose weight.

Trust me. You are going to like this.

INGREDIENTS:

- 3 corn tortillas (Read the label. There should only be corn and lime juice in the ingredients. My favorite brand is Food for Life but this can be hard to find unless you have a Whole Foods Market near you. The locally made ones are often prefect, too.)
- 1 sweet potato, cooked
- ½ cup cooked black beans (no salt or rinse before using if they contain salt)
- ½ cup cooked greens (steamed kale collards, or spinach)
- 2 green onions, sliced
- hot sauce (I love Sriracha even though it is a Korean sauce on this Mexican dish.)
- salsa (optional)
- nutritional yeast (optional. Some people love it and some people don't)
- guacamole (optional. Mash avocado, lime juice, and chili powder to taste.)

INSTRUCTIONS:

1. Warm corn tortillas in the microwave covered with a damp paper towel for a few seconds.

2. Mash the sweet potato with a fork (optional. Add ground cumin, chili powder, garlic powder, onion powder, and cayenne to taste)

3. Place onto the tortilla.

4. Top with beans, greens, and green onions, plus hot sauce, salsa, nutritional yeast and guacamole as desired.

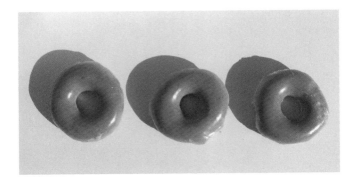

10. DONUTS! YES, I SAID DONUTS WITH FROSTING

This recipe is so sweet and decadent. You might feel a little afraid to eat it without feeling guilty, but go for it, girlfriend. It does have nuts and dried fruit so just don't eat this everyday while you are losing weight.

Every ingredient is a 100% whole food so you can eat it without guilt.

Women with PCOS should avoid soy product as they will raise the estrogen levels in the body and this is not good. For this reason you want to stay away from all the "fake" foods made with soy such as the fake meats and fake cheeses, the yogurt made with tofu, etc.

This recipe has such a small amount of tofu that I don't think you need to worry about it.

INGREDIENTS

- 5 Medjool dates, pitted and chopped
- 1/4 cup golden raisins
- 1/2 cup water
- 1-3/4 cups rolled oats
- 2 teaspoons baking powder
- 1 teaspoon baking soda
- 2 teaspoons cinnamon
- 1 teaspoon ground nutmeg
- 1/4 teaspoon ground clove
- 1/2 of a ripe banana, diced
- 1 cup almond milk
- 1-1/2 cups grated carrots
- 1/2 cup raisins
- 1/2 cup walnuts, chopped

DIRECTIONS

1. Preheat oven to 350 degrees with the rack in the center position. In a small bowl, combine the 5 dates, 1/4 cup raisins, and 1/2 cup water. Soak for 15 minutes.

2. Grind the rolled oats in a high-speed blender until it turns to flour. Mix in baking powder, soda, cinnamon,

nutmeg, and clove.

3. Transfer the soaked dates, raisins, and water to a high-speed blender and blend for 30 seconds. Add the banana and unsweetened almond or rice milk and blend until smooth.

4. Fold the wet and dry ingredients gently together.

5. Fold in the carrots, raisins, and walnuts.

6. Spoon batter into a non-stick donut pan, filling to the top.

7. Bake for 20-25 minutes.

8. Remove from oven and cool for 5-7 minutes before removing the donuts from pan. Loosen the edges with a fork to remove from pan.

FROSTING FOR DONUTS

INGREDIENTS

- 5 Medjool dates, pitted and chopped
- 1/2 cup raw cashews (not salted or roasted)
- 3/4 cup water
- 3 tablespoons lemon juice or crushed pineapple
- 1 teaspoon vanilla extract
- 2 tablespoons tofu (silken or firm) (This is such a small amount of tofu that I don't think you have to worry about the soy.)
- 1/4 cup water (plus 2-3 more tablespoons as needed)

DIRECTIONS

1. Soak the dates and cashews in 3/4 cup water for 15-30 minutes.
2. Drain water off the dates and set aside
3. Combine all ingredients in a high-speed blender.
4. Blend until very smooth, adding more water as needed to reach desired consistency.

Frost donuts before serving.

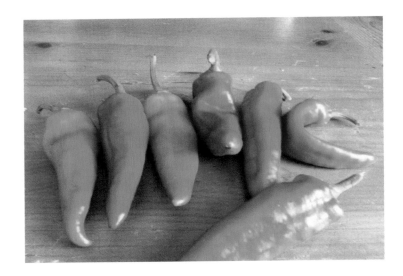

11. BORDER CROSSING TEX-MEX LASAGNA

What border are we crossing with this lasagna? We are definitely into uncharted lands.

Wait, I thought lasagna was an Italian dish. Not anymore.

I have to admit that I toss a few raisins into this dish. I love the sweet surprise every once in a while. You will learn what you like as you make these meals.

Women with PCOS often crave sugar. We can satisfy it in healthy ways and we should. Life is meant to be enjoyed.

If you enjoy your food it isn't a diet. It is pure heaven.

INGREDIENTS

Sauce:
- 2 8-ounce cans tomato sauce
- 3 cups water
- 4 tablespoons cornstarch
- 3 tablespoons chili powder
- ½ teaspoon onion powder
- ¼ teaspoon garlic powder

Place all ingredients for the sauce in a saucepan. Mix well until well combined. Cook and stir over medium heat until thickened, about 5 minutes. Taste and add more chili powder if desired. Set aside.

- 10-12 corn tortillas (Read the label. There should only be corn and lime juice.)

- 4 cups mashed pinto beans (no salt or rinse before using)

- 1 cup chopped green onions
- 1 ½ cups frozen corn kernels, thawed
- 1 can sliced ripe olives, drained (rinse to take away some of the salt)
- 1-2 tablespoons chopped green chilies (optional)

INSTRUCTIONS

Preheat oven to 350 degrees.

To assemble casserole:

Place the beans in a large bowl. Add the onions, corn, olives and green chilies. Mix well.

1. Place 1½ cups of the sauce in the bottom of a non-stick oblong baking dish.

2. Cover the bottom of the baking dish with a layer of corn tortillas.

3. Spread half of the bean mixture over the tortillas.

4. Make another layer of tortillas over the bean mixture and then spread the remaining bean mixture on top of those tortillas.

5. Cover with another layer of tortillas and then pour the remaining sauce over the tortillas.

6. Cover with parchment paper, cover with aluminum foil.

7. Bake for 45 minutes.

8. Remove from oven and let sit for about 15 minutes before cutting.

Serve with salsa

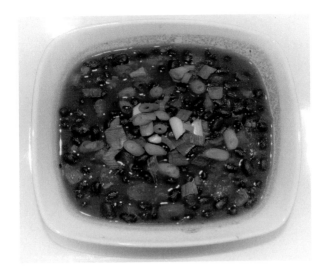

12. WINTER WARMING BLACK BEAN CHILI WITH CORN CHIPS

Long, cold, dark winter days need something that will warm us up. You will love this black bean chili comfort food. It is so simple and easy to make that it can easily become a "go to" recipe.

What is even better? The corn chips. I mean, heck, we need corn chips for snacking on once in a while, right?

When you are looking for corn tortillas at the grocery store read the labels. There should be two ingredients, corn and lime juice.

I love the Food for Life brand. They make all of their products with 100% whole and sprouted grains. HEALTHY. HEALTHY. HEALTHY.

INGREDIENTS

- 2 ½ cups vegetable broth (low salt is best)
- 1 medium onion, chopped
- 1 red bell pepper, chopped
- 3 cloves garlic, minced
- 1 4-ounce can chopped green chilies
- 1 tablespoon chili powder
- 1 teaspoon ground cumin
- 1 teaspoon oregano
- 1 15-ounce can black beans, drained and rinsed (no salt is best)
- 1 15-ounce can chopped tomatoes (low salt is best but can be hard to find)
- 2/3 cup quick cooking barley
- 3 tablespoons chopped fresh cilantro
- dash salt
- baked tortilla Chips (recipe below)
- avocado salsa (recipe below)

INSTRUCTIONS

1. Place ½ cup of the vegetable broth in a large pot. Add onions, bell pepper, and garlic. Cook and stir frequently for 3 minutes.

2. Add green chilies, chili powder, cumin, and oregano. Cook and stir for 2 minutes.

3. Add remaining broth, beans, tomatoes, and barley.

4. Bring to a boil, reduce heat, cover, and cook for 10 minutes.

5. Uncover and cook for 15 minutes. Stir in cilantro and salt to taste.

AVOCADO SALSA

Look at these ingredients. They are all whole foods.

Avocados are a good source of the good oils we need.

When you are trying to lose weight quickly you need to limit that amount of avocados you eat, even though they are a great nutritious food and you will eat plenty of them in your lifetime. Limit them for more rapid weight loss. It is not such a big deal. There are other foods that will be such a taste sensation you will not miss the avocados.

Have a tomato salsa instead but just for now. When your weight is back to normal you can have plenty of avocados.

- 2 medium avocados, peeled and diced
- 1 large, firm, ripe tomato, chopped
- 2 tablespoons finely chopped red onion
- 2 tablespoons finely chopped, seeded, jalapeno pepper
- 2 tablespoons finely chopped fresh cilantro
- 2 tablespoons fresh lime juice

Combine all ingredients and mix.

CORN TORTILLAS

These corn chips are a great snack for you because they are a 100% whole grain and there is no oil or salt.

1. Preheat oven to 350 °F and line a cookie sheet with parchment paper.

2. Cut corn tortillas into triangles and place on prepared cookie sheet.

4. Sprinkle with seasonings if desired. (I like Mrs. Dash No Salt Fiesta Blend.)

3. Bake 8-10 minutes or until crisp (They crisp as they cool).

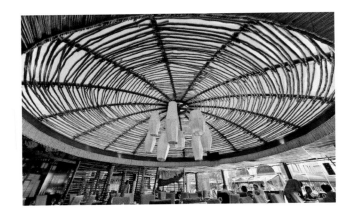

13. AFRICAN RICE ADVENTURE

This meal is all about the spices. Over time you will find the exact amounts of each spice to suit you and your family. This recipe is a good starting point. The spices turn rice and vegetables into an adventure to a far off land.

Make big pots of food that can be heated in a couple of minutes and you'll have something to eat when you get hungry.

Make big pots of brown rice too. Break it up into smaller amounts, put it into zip lock bags, and toss it into the freezer. You won't need to wait for the brown rice to cook when you make dinner after work.

INGREDIENTS

- 5 tbsp. tomato sauce
- ¼ cup vegetable broth
- 1 small onion, diced
- a dash of cinnamon
- ½ tsp cumin
- ½ tsp chili powder
- ¼ tsp mild curry powder
- 2 cups mixed frozen vegetables
- 1½ cups cooked brown rice
- hot sauce to taste

INSTRUCTIONS

1. Pour tomato sauce into a pot

2. Add broth until liquid completely covers the bottom.

3. Add onions, cinnamon, cumin, chili powder, and curry powder.

4. Saute over high heat until onions become translucent.

5. Turn heat down to low and add frozen vegetables, stirring to warm them.

6. Add cooked rice and stir to completely combine.

7. Add one more tbsp. tomato sauce, plus salt and black pepper to taste.

8. Add hot sauce to taste.

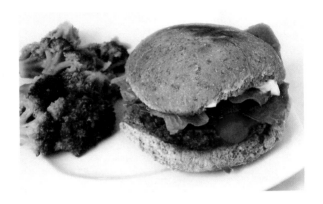

14. EVERYBODY LOVES BURGERS

Sometimes you just want a burger, a simple burger. Eating healthy rice and bean meals or potato and vegetable seems too fancy. You just want a burger.

Well, you don't have to feel deprived. I mean that. Feeling deprived will sabotage this lifestyle change. You need to feel completely satisfied or you will go back to addictive fats and sugar and salt and especially dairy.

Women with PCOS need to make a lifestyle change when it comes to food because this is not a condition that will go away. It leads to diabetes down the road.

So when you are in the mood for a burger you can make these. You will find the catchup recipe with the hash browns in chapter 3.

INGREDIENTS

- 15 ounces black beans, drained and rinsed
- 2 tbsp ketchup
- 1 tbsp yellow mustard
- 1 tsp garlic powder
- 1 tsp onion powder
- ⅓ cup instant oats

INSTRUCTIONS

1. Preheat oven to 400F. Line cookie sheet with parchment paper and set aside.

2. Mash black beans with a fork until mostly pureed

3. Stir in condiments and spices until well combined.

4. Mix in oats.

5. Divide into 4 thin patties.

6. Bake for 7 minutes

7. Flip and bake for another 7 minutes

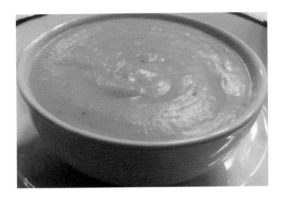

15. EPIC NO BUTTER NO NUT BUTTERNUT SOUP

Butternut squash has such a wonderful flavor. This dish is rich and creamy with a little bite to it from the chilies. I like to add a can of garbanzo beans to this soup to make it even more hearty.

You want to have recipes for foods with all different textures. I wonder if anyone has done a study on when and why we hunger for creamy foods. This soup dish will hit whatever that spot is.

A bowl of this rich soup and a nice green salad and your eyes will be feasting on the colors before your first bite.

INGREDIENTS

- 1 whole butternut squash
- 2 cups vegetable broth
- 4 ounces green chilies, diced
- 2 whole limes

INSTRUCTIONS

1. Preheat oven to 375 °F.

2. Slice squash in half (lengthwise) and place cut side down on a cookie sheet. Bake until skin is starting to brown (about 30-40 minutes).

3. Once cool enough to handle, scoop out and discard seeds. Scoop the flesh away from the skin and transfer to a blender.

4. Blend squash with broth until a smooth soup consistency.

5. Blend in green chilies.

6. Reheat the soup on low on the stove top if necessary.

7. Squeeze fresh lime juice on top before serving.

6. Reheat the soup on low on the stove top if necessary.

7. Squeeze fresh lime juice on top before serving.

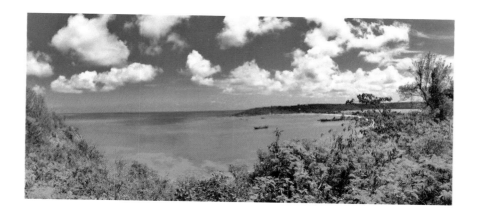

16. DREADLOCKS RASTA CARIBBEAN BLACK-EYED PEAS & RICE

Turn on a little Bob Marley and run away to a Caribbean island with this recipe.

INGREDIENTS

- 1 bunch scallions, white parts sliced thin
- 2 whole celery ribs, minced
- 4 whole garlic cloves, minced
- 2 tbsp. fresh ginger root, minced
- 4 whole fresh thyme leaves
- 1½ tsp. Tabasco green pepper sauce
- 2 tbsp. ketchup (See recipe for HASH BROWNS in chapter 3)
- ¼ tsp. turmeric (optional)
- 1 bunch kale, chopped
- 15 ounces black-eyed peas, drained and rinsed
- 1 cup brown rice, uncooked
- 2½ cups vegetable broth
- 2 tsp. Jamaican dried jerk seasoning

INSTRUCTIONS

1. Combine rice with 2 cups of vegetable broth in a large pot and set aside.

2. Line a skillet with a thin layer of vegetable broth and add scallions, celery, garlic, ginger, thyme, Tabasco green pepper sauce, and 1 tsp. jerk seasoning.

3. Cook over high heat, adding additional broth as necessary, until the celery is soft, about 3 minutes.

4. Add remaining jerk seasoning, stirring to coat.

5. Add to rice & add 2 tbsp. of ketchup and turmeric.

6. Cover and bring to a boil.

7. Once boiling, reduce heat to low and simmer 40-50 minutes until rice is cooked, adding broth as needed.

8. Meanwhile, lightly steam greens. Press out any excess water and chop into bite-sized pieces.

9. Once rice is fully cooked, fluff with a fork and then stir in black-eyed peas and greens.

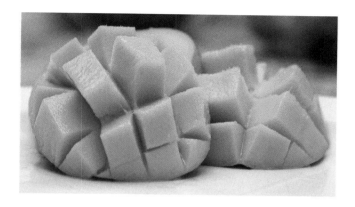

17. SIMPLE MANGO SALSA

Everyone loves mangoes. You can put this mango salsa on everything. It is great with chips of course, on potatoes, on rice, in salads, on tacos, and on burritos. I have even put it on my oatmeal in the morning and didn't regret it. I swear you could eat your shoes if they had this mango salsa on top.

INGREDIENTS

- 2 cups peeled, chopped, ripe mango
- ½ cup finely chopped onion
- ½ cup finely chopped red bell pepper
- 1 fresh jalapeno, seeded and finely chopped
- ¼ teaspoon minced fresh garlic
- 1 tablespoon cider vinegar
- 1 tablespoon warm water
- several twists freshly ground black pepper
- dash salt

INSTRUCTIONS

Combine all ingredients in a bowl and mix well. Cover and chill at least 1 hour before serving.

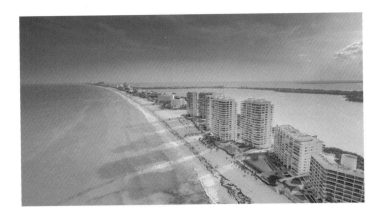

18. CANCUN SPRING BREAK CHILE RELLENOS

Many women that I work with call to say they like these chili rellenos better than the ones filled with cheese.

They are a tiny bit labor intensive the first time you try to make them because you have to roast the peppers and let them sit for 15 minutes to cool, but it is well worth the effort.

INGREDIENTS

- 4 large poblano chili peppers
- 2 cups garlic mashed potatoes
- 1 ½ cups fat-free re-fried pinto beans
- ¼ cup water
- ¼ teaspoon chipotle chili powder

INSTRUCTIONS

1. Preheat broiler.

2. Lay chilies in a single layer on a dry baking sheet.

3. Broil about 4 inches from broiler until chilies are blistering and charred on all sides, turning frequently (about 15 minutes).

4. Put chilies in a large metal bowl, cover with plastic wrap, and let sit for 15 minutes.

5. Remove skins with your hands or rub with a paper towel.

6. Set aside on paper towels to dry.

7. Place the beans, water, and chipotle powder in a small saucepan until warmed, stirring frequently. Do not boil.

8. Place 1 cup of the mixture in the bottom of a medium baking dish.

9. Preheat oven to 375 degrees.

10. Cut a slit down the side of each poblano and remove the seeds. You may leave the stem on or remove it.

11. Stuff the poblanos with about ½ cup of mashed potatoes each. Close the poblanos and place in the baking dish.

12. Top with 1 cup of the sauce.

13. Cover and bake for 20 minutes, uncover and bake about 10 more minutes.

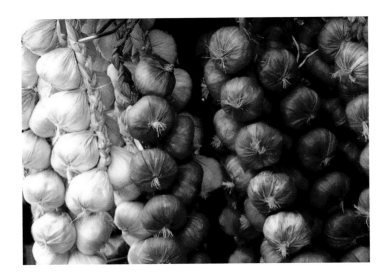

19. GARLIC MASHED POTATOES

INGREDIENTS

- 4 large Yukon Gold potatoes
- 2 cloves garlic
- ¼ cup unsweetened almond or rice milk
- several twists freshly ground white pepper
- dash sea salt (optional. Salt retains water which is not good for losing weight.)

INSTRUCTIONS

1. Peel potatoes and chop into chunks. Place in a stainless pan with water to cover.

2. Add 2 whole cloves of peeled garlic. Bring to a boil, reduce heat, cover and cook for 15 minutes until potatoes are tender.

3. Drain.

4. Mash in pan using potato masher, adding the remaining ingredients to get a smooth consistency.

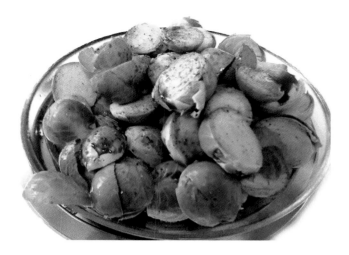

20. KID LOVIN' ROASTED BRUSSELS SPROUTS

I don't know how this recipe became a favorite for Christmas and Thanksgiving at our house. Maybe it is because the pine nuts and the caramelized onions give it a rather sweet flavor. Even the kids who swear they don't like Brussels sprouts like this recipe.

INGREDIENTS

- 1 pound Brussels sprouts
- 1 ½ cups vegetable broth
- 1 yellow onion, diced
- 2/3 cup pine nuts
- freshly ground black pepper

INSTRUCTIONS

1. Preheat oven to 400 degrees.

2. Clean Brussels sprouts.

3. Cut off the ends and cut Brussels sprouts in half.

4. Place Brussels sprouts in a bowl.

5. Pour 1 cup of the vegetable broth over the Brussels sprouts and mix with the broth.

6. Space the Brussels sprouts onto a baking sheet.

7. Bake for 40 minutes until they become brown. Remove from oven and set aside.

8. Place the onions in a non-stick sauté pan and spread out evenly.

9. Cook over medium heat.

10. Cook until onions begin to brown on the bottom.

11. Stir and spread out evenly again.

12. Place the pine nuts in a non-stick saute pan on medium heat and toast about 2 to 3 minutes until they are a light brown color.

13. Take the pan off the heat after 1 minute of cooking and shake before placing them back on the stove. Once they have turned light brown, turn off the heat.

14. Add the Brussels sprouts and toasted pine nuts to the sauté pan with the onions and adjust the heat to low.

15. Add the remaining ½ cup of vegetable broth and mix well.

16. Cook for 2 to 5 more minutes.

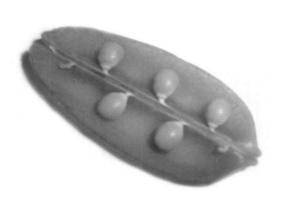

20. EASIER THAN EASY ROASTED CORN WITH SNAPPY SNAP PEAS

I suggest you make this dish while watching TV, texting, doing the laundry, cleaning your house, and taking selfies with your friends all at the same time while blindfolded. It is that easy.

Did I mention that it is also very cheap to make, too? Frozen vegetables are just as healthy for you as fresh vegetables and much less expensive. They are often even healthier for you since the vegetables are picked ripe which allows for more vitamins to form in the vegetables. Just be sure there no other ingredients in the package.

INGREDIENTS

- 3 cups frozen corn
- 3 cups frozen sugar snap peas
- 1 cup vegetable broth
- freshly ground black pepper
- 1 lime (optional)

INSTRUCTIONS

1. Preheat oven to 350 degrees.
2. Spread the frozen vegetables on to a baking sheet.
3. Pour the broth evenly over the vegetables.
4. Bake for 30 minutes.
5. Squeeze fresh lime juice over the top. (optional)

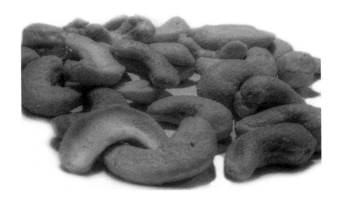

21. REALLY? ARE YOU KIDDING ME? NO CHEESE CHEESE SAUCE

Would you like mac and cheese? How about nachos with cheese? How about a burger with cheese? How about a cheese dip for vegetables? How about any vegetable in the world smothered in cheese?

You are going to love this multipurpose cheese sauce.

I have warned you in other chapters to limit the amount of nuts you are eating if you need rapid weight loss. I don't want to discourage you from eating them as they are a great whole food with good oils; just don't go nuts on nuts. Limit the amount you eat to 2 ounces for the day.

Nuts are very calorie dense which means a small amount is high in calories.

INGREDIENTS

- ¼ cup raw cashews
- 1 cup roasted butternut squash
- ¾ cup water
- 8 ounces pimientos
- ¼ cup nutritional yeast
- 3 tablespoons cornstarch

INSTRUCTIONS

1. Place all the ingredients in a blender and process until completely smooth (about 5 minutes).

2. Pour the mixture into a saucepan and cook at medium heat until the sauce thickens (about 5 minutes).

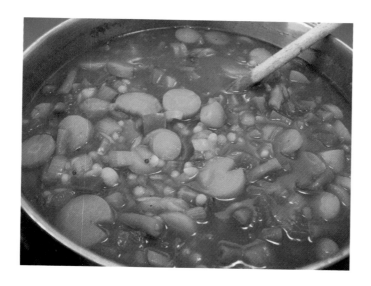

22. 15 MINUTE HEALTHY SOUPY STEWY MEAL

Throw in all the left over vegetables you have in the refrigerator. Make a big pot so you can take this with you for lunch.

INGREDIENTS

- 1 15-ounce can diced tomatoes
- 1 15-ounce can crushed tomatoes
- 2 15-ounce cans beans (Any kind you like. No salt is best or rinse before using.)
- 2 pounds frozen mixed vegetables (California Blend or Italian Blend is good.)
- 1-2 cups cooked potatoes, brown rice, or corn pasta

seasonings: minced garlic, basil, oregano, hot pepper sauce or minced garlic, grated ginger, smoked paprika, cumin, hot pepper sauce

Place all of the ingredients into a large pot and mix well. Bring to a boil and simmer for 15 minutes, until all vegetable are cooked.

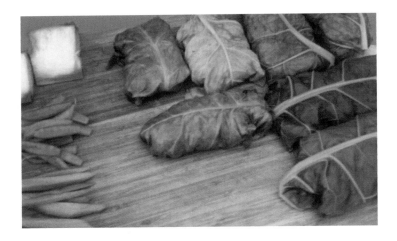

23. BEAUTIFUL CLASSY COLLARD WRAPS

You need to find a way to eat at least 2 cups of greens every day. This will nourish your blood. A lot of women start the day off with a green smoothie.

This recipe is another very classy way to eat collard greens. They are nice to take to a party, too.

INGREDIENTS

- 1 bunch collards
- 8 tablespoons hummus (see next recipe)
- 2 green onions, chopped
- 1/2 cup cilantro, chopped
- 1/4 red pepper, cut in thin strips
- 1/4 small cucumber, cut in thin strips (skin optional)
- 1/4 cup shredded carrots
- 1/2 lemon

INSTRUCTIONS

1. Put about 2 inches of water in a large frying pan and bring to a boil.

2. Lay collard greens flat and cut off the thick stem at the point where the leaf begins.

3. Place in boiling water. Cover and cook for about 2 minutes.

4. Drain and then lay flat on a board or counter, thick part of stem facing up.

5. Down the center spine of the 4 collard leaves put a row of about 2 tablespoons hummus, sprinkle with green onions, cilantro and shredded carrots. Place thin red pepper strips and cucumber strips on top.

6. Sprinkle with some lemon juice.

7. Start with the side nearest you and flip that over the filling. Turn up the end piece on the non-thick stem side

and then gently roll into a long sausage shape. Repeat until all are rolled up.

8. With a sharp knife, cut into many small pieces.

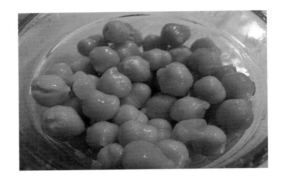

24. YUMMY HUMMUS SPREAD FOR EVERY OCCASION

Use this hummus spread in place of mayonnaise and other high fat spreads and dips.

INGREDIENTS

- 2 15-ounce cans of garbanzo beans OR cannelloni beans, 1 drained
- 3/4 to 1 cup water or the water from 1 can of beans
- 2 to 4 cloves garlic, peeled
- 4 tablespoons sesame seeds
- 2 to 4 tablespoons fresh lemon juice
- 1/4 to 1 teaspoon cumin
- 1/4 teaspoon smoked paprika
- 1/8 to 1/2 teaspoon chipotle chili powder or cayenne pepper

INSTRUCTIONS

1. Place all ingredients in the blender or food processor in the order listed, using the smaller amounts.

2. Start the machine on low and increase speed to high. (Stop and use a spatula to push it down every now and then.) If the mixture is too thick, add additional water or lemon juice a little at a time. Turn up to the highest speed and blend for a few seconds until hummus is completely smooth.

3. Stop blender and taste the hummus. Add additional seasonings to taste and blend briefly to combine.

4. Let rest for at least one hour.

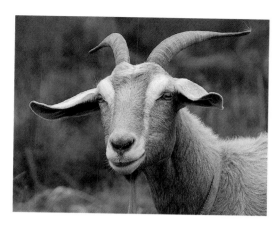

25. NO SHEPHERD NEEDED VEGETABLE PIE

Research shows that removing meat, milk, all animal products, high fat and high protein foods may reduce the risk of diabetes and even gestational diabetes. It boosts the hormone-binding proteins which help to prevent obesity.

Research also shows that eating only one egg a week may double the odds of getting diabetes.

Research also shows that fish, especially salmon, is one of the primary sources of PCBs and other industrial toxins, which may play a role in the development of diabetes.

Women with PCOS are at a very high risk of developing diabetes but you don't have to.

INGREDIENTS

- 3 cups vegetable broth
- 1 onion, chopped
- 1 stalk celery, sliced
- 1 green bell pepper, chopped
- ½ teaspoon minced bottled fresh garlic
- ½ teaspoon sage leaves
- ½ teaspoon marjoram
- 1 tablespoon soy sauce
- 1 carrot, thinly sliced
- 1 ½ cups sliced fresh mushrooms
- 1 ½ cups cauliflower florets
- 1 cup thinly sliced cabbage
- 1 cup green beans, cut in 1 inch pieces
- 2 tablespoons cornstarch mixed in 1/3 cup cold water
- freshly ground pepper to taste
- 3 cups mashed potatoes
- paprika to garnish

INSTRUCTIONS

1. Preheat oven to 350 degrees.

2. Place ½ cup of the broth in a large pot with the onion, celery, bell pepper, and garlic.

3. Cook, stirring occasionally, for about 4 minutes.

4. Stir in sage, marjoram, and soy sauce.

5. Add the remaining vegetable broth and the carrot, mushrooms, cauliflower, cabbage, and green beans.

6. Bring to a boil, cover, reduce heat, and cook for 20 minutes, stirring occasionally.

7. Add the cornstarch mixture and stir until thickened.

8. Season with pepper to taste.

9. Transfer to a casserole dish.

10. Cover vegetable mixture with mashed potatoes and sprinkle with paprika.

11. Bake for 30 minutes until potatoes are slightly browned.

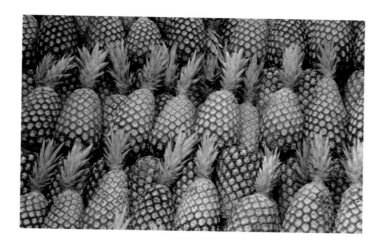

26. OH SO SWEET THAI RICE

Have you ever noticed that Thai dishes almost always have a combination of 4 flavors? They are salty, sweet, sour, and spicy. This rice dish has all these flavors.

I know you are wondering where the salt flavor comes from, as it is not listed in the ingredients. Celery brings a salty flavor without the problems related to salt such as water retention and high blood pressure.

INGREDIENTS

- 2 cups long grain brown rice
- 2-3 medium carrots
- 1 red bell pepper
- 1 green bell pepper
- 1 large onion
- 2-3 celery stalks
- 1 ½ cups broccoli
- 20 ounces canned pineapple chunks
- ¼ cup vegetable broth

INSTRUCTIONS

1. Begin by putting the rice on to cook, either in a pan or rice cooker.

2. Cut carrots in half, then cut into matchstick pieces, about 2 inches long and 1/4 to 1/8 inch thick. Cut bell peppers into ½ inch squares. Chop onion into ¼ inch pieces. Slice celery lengthwise, then into 1/8 inch thick slices. Chop broccoli into bite sized pieces, like mini trees. Set all the vegetables aside in one bowl.

3. Drain the pineapple and reserve the liquid.

4. Combine ¼ cup of the reserved pineapple juice with the vegetable broth. Set aside.

5. When the rice is within 5-10 minutes of finishing cooking, preheat a large sauté pan or wok until very hot. Add the liquid mixture (it should instantly steam and boil). Pour all of the vegetables into the pan and sauté on high,

stirring frequently.

6. When onion starts to become clear and less pungent, the vegetables are done. Add the hot cooked rice to the vegetables and mix well. Stir in the drained pineapple chunks.

7. Reduce heat to medium and continue to cook for about 5-10 minutes, adding a bit more pineapple juice to taste as desired.

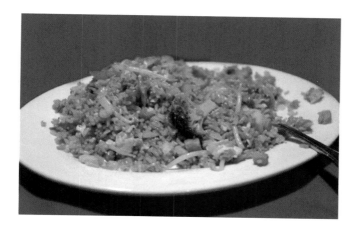

27. FRIED WITHOUT FRYING FRIED RICE

The problem with most Chinese food is all the oil and MSG used. Sure there are a lot of vegetables in the meals, which is absolutely great, but all that oil packs on the pounds.

Fried rice can be made without oil, and you should learn to make it this way because it tastes good and is an easy way to make an average meal - an over the top great meal.

Long grain brown rice is not as nutty and chewy as short grain brown rice. If you are used to eating a lot of white rice, switch to the long grain and it will feel more familiar to you and your family.

INGREDIENTS

- ¼ cup water (Vegetable broth can be substituted for more flavor.)
- ½-1 teaspoon crushed garlic (You should always have a jar of garlic in the frig.)
- ½-1 teaspoon grated ginger (You can buy this in a jar too.)
- 6 cups mixed chopped vegetables (carrots, broccoli, red peppers, green onions, celery, snow peas, bok choy (a great way to add more greens to this dish), etc.
- 4 cups cooked brown rice
- ¼ cup low sodium soy sauce (Soy products should be avoided by women with PCOS but this is a small amount.)

INSTRUCTIONS

Place the water in a wok or large non-stick frying pan. Add the garlic and ginger and heat until water boils. Add the vegetables and cook, stirring frequently, until vegetables are crisp and tender. Stir in the rice and soy sauce.

Cook until heated through, about 2 minutes.

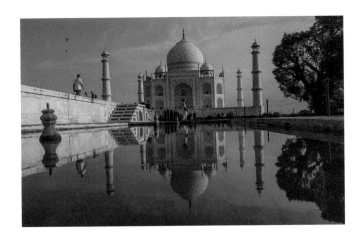

28. A BILLION PEOPLE CAN'T BE WRONG DAL

Dal is a staple food in India that has a population of 1.252 billion people. Indians have been eating dal as their main source of protein for thousands of years. Now, you are going to eat it too.

The European Association for the Study of Diabetes, the Canadian Diabetes Association, and the American Diabetes Association all recommend we eat pulses to control diabetes. But what the heck are pulses? They're dried peas, beans, and legumes.

Women with PCOS need to keep their blood sugar well-regulated which will lower the circulating androgen (male hormone). This will help to regulate your menstrual cycle and help rid you of the embarrassing excess facial hair that comes from the high levels of these hormones.

Indians eat dal on rice, but you should try it on potatoes too.

INGREDIENTS

- 2 cups split mung beans, chana dal or yellow split peas
- 5 cups water
- 1 ½ tablespoons curry powder (sweet, mild, or spicy)
- Sriracha sauce (optional)

INSTRUCTIONS

1. Place the beans or peas and the water in a medium pot. Bring to a boil, reduce heat, cover and simmer for 30 minutes.

2. Add the curry powder, mix well, and cook uncovered for 30 minutes longer.

3. Transfer to a serving bowl and let rest for about 15 minutes, to thicken slightly, before serving.

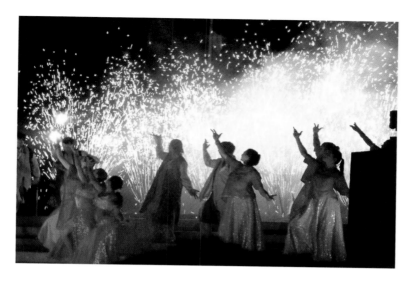

29. BOLLYWOOD BIRYANI

I was working as an acupuncturist on a cruise ship in the South Pacific. Cruise ships are known for their over the top buffets which is all well and good for most people, but I eat a whole food plant based diet with no salt, oil, or sugar.

It was slim pickings for me until I discovered the Indian vegetable biryani. Now it is time for you to sail off to a foreign land and delight in this explosive dish.

INGREDIENTS

- 1 onion, chopped
- 2 cloves garlic, crushed
- 2 ½ teaspoons curry powder
- ¾ teaspoon cinnamon
- ¼ teaspoon cloves
- 2 ¾ cups water
- 2 carrots, thinly sliced
- ½ cauliflower, broken into florets
- ½ cup raisins
- 1 cup uncooked brown rice
- 1 cup peas, fresh or frozen
- 1 tomato, chopped
- Sriracha hot sauce to taste

INSTRUCTIONS

1. In a large pan, cook onions and garlic in ¼ cup of the water for 5 minutes.

2. Add curry powder, cinnamon, and cloves, cook 2 minutes.

3. Add the remaining water, carrots, cauliflower, raisins, and rice. Bring to a boil.

4. Cover, reduce heat, and simmer about 40 minutes.

5. Stir in peas and tomatoes.

6. Cook an additional 15 minutes.

7. Top with Sriracha source to taste.

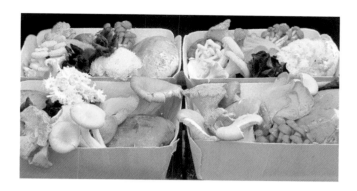

30. PILED HIGH PORTOBELLO WITH OYSTER MUSHROOMS

Portobello mushrooms marinated in balsamic vinegar are amazing. You can toss them on the grill and then put them on a 100% whole grain bun for an easy burger for tailgate parties, or for a more upscale party try this recipe.

The presentation is so beautiful you would gain extra points on Top Chef.

As you get to know your taste preferences for spices you might change this up some to suit you, but that is what you will do with all the recipes.

INGREDIENTS

- ¼ cup pearled barley
- ½ cup of water or vegetable broth
- 2 portobello mushrooms
- ¼ cup balsamic vinegar
- 1 cup oyster mushrooms, chopped
- 1 roasted red pepper
- 1 16-ounce can fire roasted chopped tomatoes
- 2 tablespoon lemon juice
- ½ teaspoon freshly ground black pepper
- 2 cloves garlic, minced
- 1 teaspoon capers
- 2 green onions, sliced
- 2 tablespoons fresh tarragon leaves
- ½ teaspoon crushed red pepper (optional)

INSTRUCTIONS

1. Place the water or broth in a small saucepan and bring to a boil. Add the barley, reduce heat, cover and cook until tender, about 35 minutes.

2. Meanwhile, remove the stems and gills from the portobello mushrooms. Set aside.

3. Place the roasted red pepper, tomatoes, lemon juice, and pepper in a food processor and process until smooth.

4. Transfer to a saucepan and add the garlic, capers, green onions, tarragon, and optional red pepper for more heat. Simmer over medium heat while cooking the mushrooms.

5. Place the oyster mushrooms in a large non-stick skillet and sear over medium heat until they brown. Remove and set aside.

6. Reduce heat to medium, add the portobellos and the balsamic vinegar. Cook gently, until the portobellos just begin to soften and sweat, adding tiny amounts of water to keep the vinegar from burning.

7. You can add a little salt to taste after cooking.

To serve:
Place the portobellos on individual plates, gill(less) side up. Divide the cooked barley into each mushroom, top with the seared oyster mushrooms, and ladle the sauce over the top.

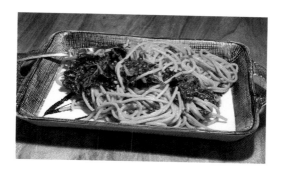

31. PASTA SUPREME FOR SUPREME WEIGHT LOSS

Have you been told to avoid pasta to lose weight? I know I was. The low carb craze has scared us all, but if it is so great why are Americans and the rest of the world for that matter getting bigger and bigger as they eat more and more meat? If it was such a great diet why isn't it working?

It is true that regular processed pasta is a big problem for people with weight problems, diabetes, and for women with PCOS.

What makes this pasta dish different is that it is made with 100% WHOLE GRAIN pasta. Whole grains will not spike your blood sugar. It is also very difficult to over eat whole grains because they are filled with fiber which is bulky in the stomach, making you feel full before you are able to over eat.

Try different types of whole grain pasta such as corn pasta, rye pasta, and different brands of whole grain pasta to find one that you like.

The 365 house brand at Whole Foods is really nice. It has a good flavor and holds together nicely which can be a problem with some brands of whole grain pastas.

The 365 brand at Whole Paycheck, I mean Whole Foods, is also priced for people on a regular budget too.

INGREDIENTS

- 2 cups vegetable broth
- 2 cups walnut pieces
- 4 tablespoons freshly parsley, chopped
- 4 tablespoons fresh cilantro, chopped
- 2 ½ teaspoons fresh lemon juice
- 1 ½ teaspoons fresh garlic, minced
- ¼ teaspoon salt (optional)
- several twists freshly ground black pepper
- dash or two of cayenne pepper (optional)
- 1 pound package uncooked pasta (made from brown rice, corn, quinoa or spelt, if you cannot handle 100% whole wheat which is true of many women with PCOS)
- 3 cups broccoli pieces
- 2 cups mixed bell pepper strips

INSTRUCTIONS

1. Place broth, walnuts, parsley, cilantro, lemon juice, garlic, salt, and pepper into a blender jar. Process until smooth. Set aside.

2. Bring a large pot of water to a boil.

3. Add pasta and cook for about 6 minutes.

4. Add broccoli and bell peppers and cook until vegetables and pasta are tender, another 4-6 minutes.

5. Remove from heat. Drain and place in a large bowl.

6. Pour sauce over and toss well to mix.

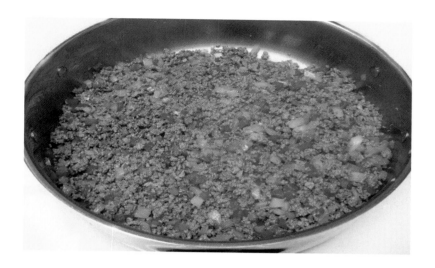

32. IT'S WEDNESDAY, IT MUST BE SLOPPY JOE'S

Human beings are creatures of habit even when it comes to what we eat. We all have about 6 meals that we choose from.

Is this familiar? "Honey, do you want chicken or meat loaf for dinner?"

We don't pick from the hundreds of thousands of choices available to us.

With this lifestyle change, you will find the dishes you like and eat those over and over. Every Wednesday I seem to have sloppy joe's. I didn't plan it this way but for some unknown reason when Wednesday rolls around, I want sloppy joe's.

I wonder what your 6 meals will turn out to be. Don't you?

INGREDIENTS

- 3 1/3 cups water
- 1 onion, chopped
- 1 green bell pepper, chopped
- 1 tablespoon chili powder
- 1 ½ cups dried brown lentils
- 1 15-ounce can crushed tomatoes
- 2 tablespoons soy sauce
- 2 tablespoons prepared mustard
- 2 tablespoons pure maple syrup (This is a whole plant based food.)
- 1 teaspoon rice vinegar
- 1 teaspoon vegetarian Worcestershire sauce
- freshly ground black pepper

INSTRUCTIONS

1. Place 1/3 cup of the water in a large pot. Add the onions, bell pepper, and maple syrup, and cook stirring occasionally until onions soften slightly, about 5 minutes.

2. Add the chili powder and mix in well.

3. Add the remaining water, the lentils, tomatoes, and the rest of the seasonings.

4. Mix well, bring to a boil, reduce heat, cover and cook over low heat for 55 minutes, stirring occasionally.

Serve on 100% whole grain. Try corn bread, rye bread, spelt bread, or whatever whole grain bread you like, or serve this on brown rice or potatoes.

Hint:
Read the labels on all breads. It should never just say "wheat". If wheat is in the bread it should say "whole wheat."

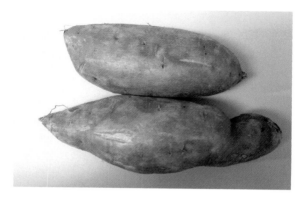

33. BLOW YOUR SOCKS OFF BAKED YAMS WITH PEANUT SAUCE

This recipe is well worth falling in love with. There is so much flavor and richness you will never want boring greasy butter ruining your yams ever again.

INGREDIENT

- Garnet Yams (reddish skins and a deep orange flesh)

INSTRUCTIONS

1. Preheat oven to 350 degrees.

2. Scrub the yams and cut into large pieces

3. Place in a single layer in a dry baking dish, skin side down.

4. Cover with parchment paper, then cover the baking dish with aluminum foil, crimping it over the sides to hold in the steam.

5. Bake for 1 hour, 10 minutes.

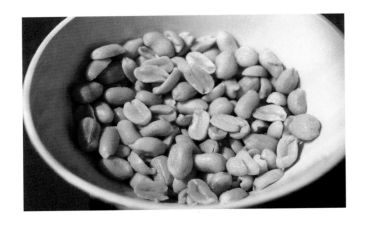

TOP WITH PEANUT DRESSING

PEANUT DRESSING

- ¾ cup rice vinegar
- ¼ cup soy sauce
- 2 tablespoons Sambal chili paste
- ¾ cup natural peanut butter (read label. There should be one ingredient. Peanuts)
- ¼ cup warm water
- 1/8 cup cilantro leaves

INSTRUCTIONS

1. Place vinegar, soy sauce and chili paste into a blender jar.

2. Process on low until mixed.

3. Add the peanut butter ¼ cup at a time and process until very smooth.

4. Add the warm water and the cilantro leaves and process until well mixed.

This recipe is well worth falling in love with. There is so much flavor and richness you will never want boring, greasy butter ruining your yams ever again.

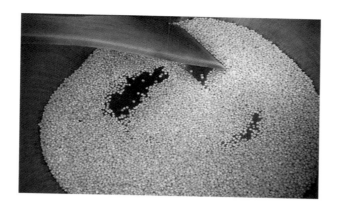

34. NOBODY THINKS OF BAKED MILLET

Millet is a very important grain in Africa and India, but here in the US people think of it as the main ingredient in bird food.

Traditional Chinese Medicine has picked up on the medicinal and healing properties of millet. It is a great grain for women with fertility problems and for women with PCOS.

Millet is not just for birds anymore.

INGREDIENTS

- 1 ¼ cups millet
- 4 cups tomato juice
- 1 onion, coarsely chopped
- 2 cloves garlic
- ½ teaspoon sage
- ½ teaspoon basil
- ½ teaspoon poultry seasoning

INSTRUCTIONS

1. Preheat oven to 350 degrees.

2. Place the millet in a large bowl.

3. Put the remaining ingredients in a blender jar and process until smooth.

4. Add to millet and mix well.

5. Pour into a square baking dish, cover, and bake for 1 ¼ hours.

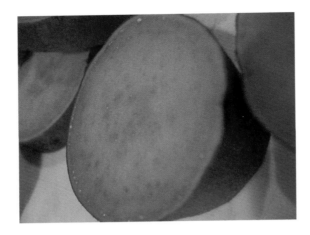

35. OUT OF THIS WORLD SPICY YAM STEW

There are many varieties of yams. They come in red, yellow, and even black. They also come in all different sizes. The yams grown in Tonga in the South Pacific can grow up to 3 feet long. You should explore them all.

In Traditional Chinese Medicine we use a Chinese yam (shan yao) in many formulas for women's fertility. It is always better to eat the yam to stay healthy, rather than waiting to become out of balance and needing to use it as medicine.

Yams are considered to be the most nutritious food on the plant. NASA, the U.S. space program, takes them into space so I guess you can say they are "out of this world," too.

INGREDIENTS

- 1 ½ cups vegetable broth
- 2 medium-large yams, peeled and chunked
- 3 stalks celery, sliced
- 1 bell pepper, chopped
- 1 onion, chopped
- 2 carrots, chopped
- 1 16-ounce can chopped tomatoes (roasted are best)
- 2 tablespoons chopped green chilies
- 2 tablespoons soy sauce (This recipe serves 8, so you will only have a small amount of soy per serving.)
- 1/4 teaspoon ground cinnamon
- ¼ teaspoon red pepper flakes
- several twists freshly ground black pepper
- 2 tablespoons cornstarch mixed in 1/3 cup cold water
- 1/3 cup fresh parsley, chopped

INSTRUCTIONS

1. Place all the ingredients (except the cornstarch mixture and the parsley) in a large pot.

2. Bring to a boil, reduce heat and cover, cook over medium-low heat for 30 minutes, or until vegetables are tender, stirring occasionally.

3. Add the cornstarch mixture and stir until thickened.

4. Stir in the parsley just before serving.

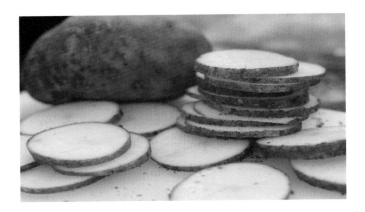

36. CRISPY CRUNCHY LIP SMACKING POTATO CHIPS

If I am not craving something sweet, I am craving some kind of "chippy" thing.

Remember, I told you that you are not allowed to feel deprived when it comes to food. There is plenty of food around and there is no reason to feel deprived, ever. Never ever, ever let yourself feel deprived.

When you are in the mood for something crispy, make a batch of these potato chips. They are completely fine to eat. They are a whole food with no oil, very little salt, and no sugar.

INGREDIENTS

- 1 large russet potato
- Salt and/or pepper to taste

INSTRUCTIONS

1. Fill a medium bowl with water and peel the potato.

2. Use a mandolin slicer on the thinnest setting, slice the potatoes. (Be careful with the mandolin. I am not the only one to slice the tip of my finger off making potato chips.)

3. Place the sliced potatoes in the bowl of water to prevent browning and remove excess starch.

4. Dry potato chips thoroughly with paper towel.

5. Line two large plates with a sheet of parchment paper and place enough potato slices on it to cover (about 9). Do not overlap.

6. Mix salt, pepper, and any other seasonings together in a bowl and sprinkle seasonings very lightly over the chips.

7. Microwave one plate of chips at a time, on high, for 3-6 minutes. Watch them for 3-4 minutes and stop the microwave when they turn a golden brown in the center.

8. Use oven mitts to remove the plate from the microwave and let cool a few minutes.

9. Remove the chips and set aside in a bowl or dish and repeat until all of your potatoes have been turned into chips.

10. Chips will crisp after they cool.

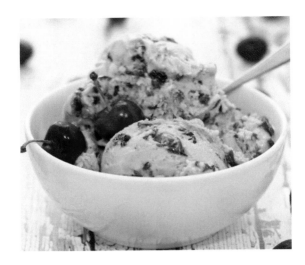

37. LAST BUT NOT LEAST CHOCOLATE CHERRY ICE CREAM

Can you believe you can have chocolate cherry ice cream? Well, yes you can. If you are an ice cream lover like me, you will love this.

I am only giving you one dessert recipe in this recipe book. I have so many good dessert recipes that I will have to make a whole recipe book just for the desserts.

INGREDIENTS

- 1/2 cup unsweetened almond milk
- 1 tbsp. cocoa or cacao powder
- 1 large ripe frozen banana (Ripe bananas have a lot of brown spots. Peel and put them in a zip lock bag, then smash it before placing into the freezer.)
- 1 cup frozen pitted cherries

DIRECTIONS

1. Place ingredients into a blender (in order listed).

2. Blend the ingredients on medium low to medium speed. Blend until smooth and cocoa is evenly distributed. (You will be shocked. When it's done it will look like ice cream, feel like ice cream, and taste amazing.)

3. Serve immediately.

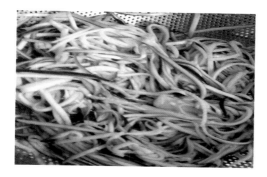

38. MARINARA WITH ZUCCHINI NOODLES

Zucchini noodles are a great option when you want to avoid wheat noodles.

Ingredients:

- ¼ cup water
- 1 yellow onion, diced
- 1 medium red bell pepper, diced
- 1 medium yellow bell pepper, diced
- 8-10 mushrooms (sliced)
- 2 cans diced or crushed no-salt tomatoes (14.5 oz. each)
- 1 small can tomato paste
- 1 teaspoon garlic powder (or 1-2 cloves minced)
- 1 ½ teaspoons dried Italian spices
- 6 medium zucchini cut finely into "noodles"
- 1/3 cup chopped fresh basil

Directions

Saute the onion in the water on medium-high heat until soft, about 2-3 minutes.

Add the bell pepper and mushrooms, and sauté 5 minutes on medium heat to soften (adding water as needed to prevent sticking).

Add the crushed tomatoes, tomato paste, garlic powder and spices, and turn down to simmer for 20 to 30 minutes.

Zucchini Noodles- Cut the ends off the zucchini first. Using a mandolin slicer, use the appropriate blade insert to create thin strings (like long matchsticks). For short noodles, cut the zucchini in half before slicing. The zucchini cooks down, so make a bunch. Place noodles into a pot of boiling water and cook for about 5 to 10 minutes until zucchini is softened (but not breaking apart).

Drain zucchini and combine with the sauce. Add the basil to the sauce and simmer for 5 minutes before serving.

Serve with grated walnuts on top. Use a rotary style cheese grater.

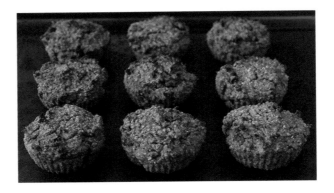

39. PUMPKIN RAISIN MUFFINS

Ingredients:

- 2 large, very ripe bananas
- ½ cup nondairy milk
- 1 15 ounce can pumpkin (not pumpkin pie filling)
- ½ cup date paste (recipe below)
- 2 tablespoons ground flax seeds
- 1 tablespoon Pumpkin Pie Spice
- 1 tablespoon Alcohol-free Vanilla
- 1 cup raisins
- 3 cups gluten-free oats

Preparation:

Preheat oven to 350 degrees F.
In a food processor fitted with the "S" blade, process bananas and nondairy milk until smooth.
Add pumpkin, date paste, flax seeds, extract, and spice and continue processing until smooth and creamy.
Transfer to a large bowl and stir in the oats and raisins.

Spoon an equal amount of batter into a muffin tin lined with cupcake liners or silicone baking cups.
Fill each muffin liner with about ½ cup of batter
Bake 45 minutes.

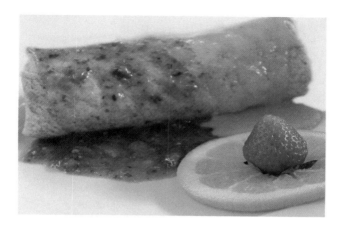

40. MEXICAN PICADILLO WRAPS

Eating about one cup of beans/legumes are recommended a day to help regulate the blood sugar levels. This is a great easy option to choose.

Ingredients:

- ½ cup water
- 1 onion, chopped
- 1 red bell pepper, chopped
- 1 teaspoon minced garlic
- 2 15 ounce cans pinto beans, drained and rinsed
- 1 14.5 ounce can fire-roasted chopped tomatoes
- 1 4 ounce can diced green chilies
- 1 tart green apple, cored and chopped
- freshly ground black pepper
- 2 cups cooked long grain brown rice
- ½ cup raisins
- 12.2 ounce can sliced black olives, drained
- ¼ cup chopped fresh cilantro
- 2 tablespoons toasted slivered almonds (optional)
- 8 - 10 Whole grain tortilla

Preparation:

Place the water into a large pot.
Add the onion, bell pepper and garlic.
Cook, stirring occasionally until onion softens slightly, about 5 minutes.
Add the beans, tomatoes, green chilies, apple and freshly ground black pepper.
Bring to a boil, reduce heat, cover and cook for 20 minutes on low.
Add the remaining ingredients, mix well and cook for 5 minutes until heated through.

Serve rolled up in a tortilla with some hot sauce sprinkled over the top

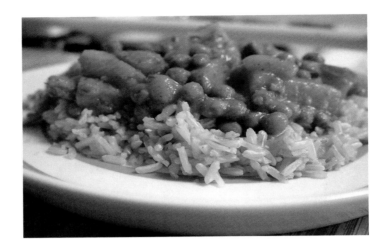

41. CREAMY VEGETABLE CURRY

Most creamy curry dishes are made with coconut milk. The saturated fat in coconut milk is not good for you. You can use soy, rice or almond milk and a bit of coconut extract.

INGREDIENTS

- 1 ¾ cups vegetable broth
- 1 onion, chopped
- 2 carrots, sliced
- 1 teaspoon minced garlic
- 2 tablespoons curry powder
- 1 teaspoon ground coriander
- ¼ teaspoon cayenne (optional)
- 2 cups chunked Yukon gold potatoes
- 2 cups green beans in 1 inch pieces
- 1 15 ounce can chopped tomatoes
- 1 15 ounce can garbanzo beans, drained and rinsed
- ½ cup frozen peas, thawed
- ½ cup unsweetened soy, rice or almond milk
- 1/8 teaspoon coconut extract

Preparation

Place ¼ cup of the broth in a large non-stick pot
Add the carrots, onions and garlic.
Cook, stirring occasionally until onion has softened, about 5 minutes.
Stir in the curry powder, coriander and cayenne (if using).
Add the remaining broth, the potatoes, beans, tomatoes and garbanzos.
Bring to a boil, reduce heat, cover and cook over low heat for about 40 minutes
Add the peas and cook for an additional 5 minutes, or until all vegetables are tender.
Mix the coconut extract into the soy, rice or almond milk.
Add to the vegetable mixture and stir well to mix.
Serve over brown basmati rice.

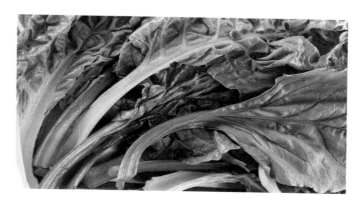

42. REALLY TASTY STEAMED CHARD

Warning: You might want to doubled, or tripled the amount you prepare as you will love the leftovers cold or hot.

Ingredients:

3 bunches Swiss chard (about 2 pounds)
1/8 to ¼ cup almond meal
¼ teaspoon garlic powder
dash sea salt
several twists freshly ground pepper
Clean the chard, remove stems, and coarsely chop.

Preparation:

Place in a steamer basket over boiling water and steam for about 3 minutes. (If you decide to use the stems as well, place the chopped stems in the steamer basket first and steam for 2 minutes before adding the chard leaves.)
Remove from steamer and drain well. Place in a large bowl.
Add 1/8 cup almond meal and the remaining seasonings and toss well to mix.
Taste and add a bit more almond meal if you'd like a richer flavor.

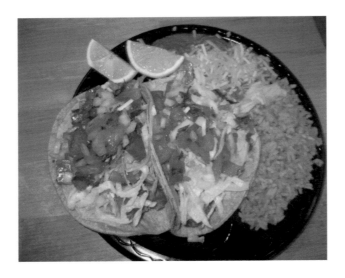

43. POTATO TACOS

Ingredients:
- 2 pounds Yukon Gold potatoes
- 1-2 teaspoons taco seasoning mix
- 4-6 tortillas
- fresh salsa
- chopped cilantro
- sliced avocado

Preparation:
Boil or microwave the potatoes with the skins on.
Cool and cube.
Place dry into a non-stick saute pan and cook until nicely browned on all sides.
Add some taco seasoning to taste, toss well and add a few drops of water to moisten seasoning if needed.
Cover and cook for another minute.
Serve on a warmed tortilla, with fresh salsa, chopped cilantro and a few slices if fresh avocado, if desired. Roll up and eat.

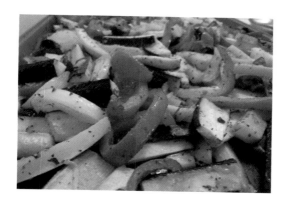

44. ROASTED VEGETABLES AND PASTA

This pasta dish has a very light sauce. The roasted vegetables give it the amazing flavor. Use 100% Whole wheat pasta if you can handle wheat or use one of the many other pastas such as corn pasta.

Ingredients:

- 1 12-ounce package of whole grain linguini or fettuccini pasta
- 3 ears of corn
- 2 zucchinis
- 1 red bell pepper
- 2 cloves of garlic, minced
- ¼ cup water
- 2 cans of unsalted chopped tomatoes
- 1 bouquet garni
- Ground black pepper and sea salt to taste, if desired

Preparation:
Preheat the oven to 350 degrees.
Place the corn, with husks still intact, zucchinis and red bell pepper directly on the baking rack.
Turn the vegetables a few times as they cook in the oven for 25 minutes.
Cook the linguine or fettuccine according to package directions. Drain, rinse with cold water and set aside.
In a non-stick pan, add the water and garlic and sauté over medium heat for 5 minutes.
Add the Pomi tomatoes (or 2 cans of unsalted) and mix well. Reduce to low heat.
Once the vegetables are finished roasting, peel the husks off the corn and cut the corn off the cob. Cut the zucchinis length-wise and chop. Cut the red bell pepper into strips and cut in half.
Add the vegetables to the garlic and tomatoes, along with the bouquet garni. Mix well.
Add the pasta and mix well. Serve with ground black pepper and sea salt to taste, if desired.

Bouquet Garni (fresh herb bundle):

Take a few fresh parsley stalks, thyme sprigs and bay leaves. Tie together with unwaxed kitchen string.
Add the bundle to the pot and remove after cooking.

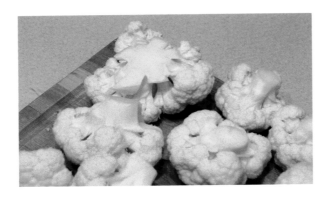

45. CAULIFLOWER COCKTAIL PARTY

This is a great choice to bring to a cocktail party. You can cook the cauliflower a day or 2 before.

Ingredients
- 3 quarts water
- 1/2 cup Old Bay Seasoning mix
- 1 onion, quartered
- 3 whole peeled garlic cloves
- ¼ cup lemon juice
- 1 large head cauliflower, cut into 1 inch florets
- Cocktail sauce, chilled (read the ingredients on label. spice it up with horseradish and vegan Worcestershire sauce to taste)

Preparation
Place the water in a large pot and add the seasoning mix, onion, garlic cloves and lemon juice.
Bring to a boil, reduce heat and simmer at a low boil for 10 minutes.
Remove onions and garlic from broth with a slotted spoon and discard.
Return liquid to a boil.
Add cauliflower, turn off heat, cover and let rest for 8-10 minutes. (don't over cook) Drain at once and spread cauliflower in a single layer on a rimmed baking sheet and let cool for a few minutes on the counter.
Place uncovered in refrigerator to finish cooling. Serve with chilled cocktail sauce to dip the cauliflower florets into before popping into your mouth.

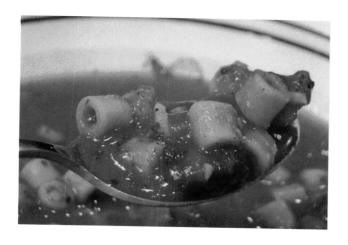

46. MINESTRONE

INGREDIENTS

- ½ cup dried kidney beans, picked over, rinsed, and soaked
- ½ cup dried great northern or cannelloni beans, picked over, rinsed, and soaked
- 6 cups water
- 8 to 10 large tomatoes, finely chopped, or 1 can (28 ounces) unsalted diced tomatoes
- 1 onion, chopped
- 4 celery stalks, chopped
- 3 carrots, chopped
- ¼ head Napa or green cabbage, chopped (you can use any greens you like. If you use spinach add at the end as they only take about 2 minutes to cook)
- ½ cup cut green beans, fresh or frozen
- 2 tablespoons vegetable broth powder
- 2 garlic cloves, minced
- 4 ounces whole wheat pasta shells, elbow macaroni, or other small pasta
- 2 tablespoons chopped fresh parsley

Preparation:

Drain the beans and put them in a large soup pot.
Add the water and bring to a boil over medium-high heat. Decrease the heat to medium-low, cover, and cook for 1 hour. Stir in the tomatoes, onion, celery, carrots, cabbage, green beans, vegetable broth powder and garlic.
Cover and cook, stirring occasionally, for about 30 minutes, until the beans and vegetables are tender.
Stir in the pasta and cook until tender, about 10 minutes. Stir in the parsley.

Serve hot.

Variation: Substitute up to 1 cup of chopped kale, spinach, or turnip greens for the cabbage. If you use fresh spinach, it will only take 1 to 2 minutes to cook. To avoid overcooking, stir in the spinach after the pasta is cooked.

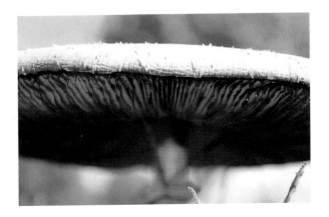

47. PORTOBELLO POOR BOY SANDWICH

INGREDIENTS

- 2 large portobello mushrooms, stemmed
- ¼ cup balsamic vinegar
- 2 to 4 tablespoons water
- 2 roasted red peppers, drained
- 2 ounces spinach leaves
- 1 small loaf whole wheat French bread, split lengthwise and halved crosswise
- 1 tablespoon low-sodium soy sauce (optional)

PREPARATION

Put the mushrooms and vinegar in a medium bowl and marinate for about 20 minutes.

Put the marinated mushrooms and 2 tablespoons of the water in a medium skillet and cook over medium heat for about 10 minutes, or just until softened and tender.

As the mushrooms cook, add more water if necessary, to prevent sticking, loosening them with a spatula.

Top each mushroom with a roasted pepper.

Cover the skillet, decrease the heat to low, and cook for 3 to 5 minutes, or until the peppers are warmed through.

SERVE

Divide the spinach leaves and put them on the bottom 2 pieces of the 100% WHOLE GRAIN bread French bread.

Cut the mushrooms and peppers in half and divide between the sandwiches.

Sprinkle with the soy sauce, if desired, and top with the remaining pieces of bread.

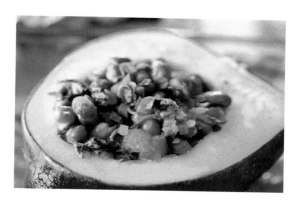

48. STUFFED ACORN SQUASH

INGREDIENTS

- ½ cup quinoa
- ½ cup diced onion
- 1½ cups diced mushrooms
- 1 cup diced celery
- ½ cup finely chopped cabbage
- ½ teaspoon sea salt
- freshly ground black pepper

PREPARATION

Preheat the oven to 375°F.
Halve the squash laterally through the center and remove seeds.

Place the squash in an 8×8-inch baking dish with the cut side down, and fill the baking dish with ¼ inch of water.

Loosely cover with foil and bake until the squash and edible skin are totally soft, about 35 minutes. Set aside.

Combine the quinoa and 1 cup of water in a small pot and bring to a boil over high heat.
Reduce the heat to low, cover, and simmer for 15 to 20 minutes, Remove the pot from the heat and let it cool, then fluff the quinoa with a fork.

Preheat a large skillet over medium heat for about 1 minute.

Add the onions and sauté for about 7 minutes, stirring often until the onions turn nice and brown.
Add water 1 to 2 tablespoons at a time, to keep the onions from sticking to the pan.

Add the mushrooms, celery, cabbage, salt, and pepper to taste, and cook for 5 more minutes, stirring occasionally.

Add the vegetable mixture to the quinoa and stir together.

Fill each of the cooked squash halves with the quinoa mixture, packing them firmly.

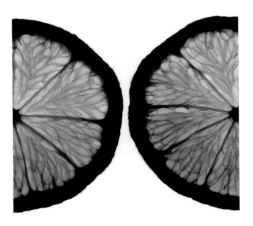

49. TOSTADAS WITH CHILI-LIME COLESLAW

Ingredients

Lentil taco "meat"

- 1 Pound of dried lentils (green or black, not red)
- 4 cups water
- 10 ounces of sliced mushrooms
- 10 ounces of chopped onion
- 4 teaspoons roasted cumin
- One tablespoon oregano
- 2 Tablespoons Chili Powder
- 2 Tablespoons salt-free seasoning
- 6 cloves garlic, pressed

Preparation

Place all ingredients in the Instant Pot electric pressure cooker on high and cook for 8 minutes or put in a pot and follow the cooking time instructions on the lentils package.

CHILI-LIME SLAW

Ingredients

Shredded cabbage
Lime juice
1/2 teaspoon crushed red pepper flakes (optional)

Preparation

Pour lime juice and red pepper flakes over shredded cabbage and let marinate at least 15 minutes before serving. Drain excess liquid before topping the tostadas.

BAKED TORTILLA CHIPS

Be sure to read the ingredients on the tortillas package. It should say "corn" or "corn and lime".

Ingredients

- Corn tortillas

Preparation

Preheat oven to 400.
Cut each tortilla into fourths.
Place on a cookie sheet covered with parchment paper.
Lightly spray each chip with water.
Sprinkle with herbs or salt-free seasonings (optional)
Bake for 10 minutes.
Turn chips over and lightly spray again with water. Bake another 8-10 minutes until crisp.

SWEET PEA GUACAMOLE

This is the prefect alternative to avocado guacamole which is high in fat.

Ingredients

- 1 – 16 ounce bag of frozen peas, defrosted
- 3 firm Roma tomatoes, diced
- One bunch of cilantro, chopped
- 1 jalapeño pepper, seeded and finely diced
- 1 shallot finely diced
- 2 cloves garlic, minced
- Juice of one lime, or more to taste
- Pinch of roasted cumin

Preparation

In a food processor fitted with the "S" blade, process peas until smooth. Stir in remaining ingredients by hand. Chill.

Assemble Tostadas

Take one tortilla and lightly swipe with sweet pea guacamole.
Heap on the lentil "meat" and top with the chili lime slaw.
Garnish with chopped cilantro or chopped scallions, if desired.

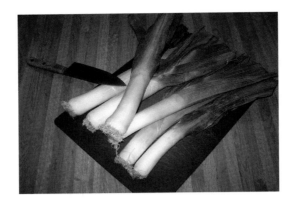

50. LEEK AND SWEET POTATO BISQUE

INGREDIENTS

3 medium sweet potatoes (about 2¼ lbs total)
3 large leeks, white and light green parts only
5-6 c unsweetened almond milk
¼ tsp nutmeg (more or less to taste)
¼ tsp ground ginger (more or less to taste)
stevia (liquid or powder) to taste (optional)

PREPARATION

Scrub sweet potatoes, then poke each a few times with a knife.

Cut each sweet potato in half and arrange in a single layer in a large microwave-safe casserole dish.

Bake at 350°F for 1–1½ hours until centers are tender when pierced with a fork.

While sweet potatoes are cooking, cut the base and green top off each leek. Slice leeks lengthwise and rinse thoroughly between layers. Then slice leeks across the grain into half-inch semicircles.

Cook the leeks in a large pot over medium heat for 5 minutes, stirring every minute or so. If leeks beginning to stick, add a little water.

Reduce heat to low and continue cooking leeks, covered, for another 20 minutes. Stir every 2–3 minutes and add a little water (1–2 Tbsp) as needed to prevent sticking.

Remove pot from heat and scoop flesh from sweet potatoes (no skin) into the pot with the leeks.

Add 4 c unsweetened almond milk, nutmeg, and ginger to pot. Blend until smooth using an immersion blender if you have one. (You can use a blender but only fill the blender half way so that it doesn't fly out of the blender and return the mixture to the pot to add the next ingredients).

Add another 1–2 cups of almond milk until soup is creamy. Sweeten to taste with stevia (optional).

Warm over low heat if needed, stirring continuously.
Serve hot with a sprinkle of nutmeg.

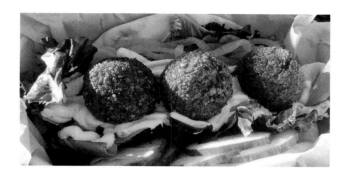

51. BAKED FALAFEL PITA SANDWICHES

Ingredients for Falafel

- 1 19oz can of garbanzo bean wash and drained
- 2 tbsp of whole wheat flour
- 1 tbsp of garlic minced
- 1 tbsp of parsley
- 1 tsp of cilantro
- 1 tsp of cumin
- 1/4 tsp of red pepper flakes
- 1 tsp of lemon juice
- 1/4 cup of onion chopped
- 1 tsp of baking powder

Ingredients for Pita sandwich

- 4 thin slices of cucumber
- 1/4 cup of fresh spinach
- 1 pita cut in half
- 1 tbsp of hummus (There are several recipes in this book)

PREPARATION

Preheat oven to 400

Combine all ingredients for falafel in a food processor and process until all ingredients are shopped and mixed together.
Return mixture to a large mixing bowl and using your hands form falafel patties.

Place patties on a greased baking sheet and bake for 15 minutes on each side or until golden brown

Cool for 5 to 10 minutes

Cut pita (Food For Life brand is pure and completely whole grain) in half place in warm oven for 2- 3 minutes to warm and make pita bread more pliable to work with.
Remove Pita from oven and spread hummus in the inside of the pita, stuff with 3 falafel patties, cucumber slices, and fresh spinach

52. SAUCES AND DRESSINGS

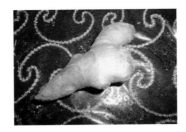

GINGER DRESSING

This dressing is excellent on any salad but don't hesitate to try in on potatoes or any vegetables.

I think having a few go-to sauces makes all the difference. Anything tastes good if you like the sauce.

INGREDIENTS

- 1/3 cup chopped red onion
- ¼ cup rice vinegar
- ¼ cup water
- 3 tablespoons grated fresh ginger
- 2 tablespoons ketchup
- 2 tablespoons soy sauce
- ½ teaspoon crushed garlic

PREPARATION

Place all ingredients in a blender or food processor and process until very smooth. Pour into a covered container and refrigerate until needed.

CILANTRO-GARLIC AIOLI

INGREDIENTS

- 1 ½ cups tofu sour cream
- 2 large cloves garlic, peeled and coarsely chopped
- juice of 1 lime
- 1/3 cup cilantro leaves
- dash salt

Place all ingredients in a food processor and process until smooth.

Keeps in refrigerator for about 2 weeks.

ASIAN PEANUT SAUCE

- ½ cup natural chunky peanut butter
- ½ cup water
- 2 tablespoons hoisin sauce
- 1 tablespoon soy sauce
- ½ tablespoon agave nectar
- 2 teaspoons chili garlic sauce
- 2 teaspoons tomato paste
- 1 teaspoon lime juice
- ½ teaspoon grated fresh ginger

Place all ingredients in a food processor and process briefly until well combined but not smooth. Pour into a covered container and refrigerate until ready to use.

WARNING: This is a higher-fat choice because of the peanut butter, so use sparingly.

BERRY VINAIGRETTE

Ingredients:

2 cups fresh or frozen strawberries or raspberries
4 tablespoons red wine vinegar
2 teaspoons agave
freshly ground pepper to taste

Instructions:

Place all ingredients in a food processor or blender. Process until smooth.

AGAVE MUSTARD DRESSING

Ingredients:

- 1/2 cup rice vinegar
- 1/2 cup balsamic vinegar
- 1/3 cup agave
- 3 tablespoons Dijon mustard
- freshly ground pepper to taste

Instructions:

Place all ingredients in a blender and process until smooth

TOFU ISLAND DRESSING

INGREDIENTS

- 1 12.3- ounce package firm silken tofu
- 1/3 cup water
- 1 tablespoon lemon juice
- 3 tablespoons ketchup
- 2 tablespoons sweet pickle relish
- 1 tablespoon minced parsley
- 1 tablespoon minced red onion
- 1 teaspoon soy sauce
- several twists fresh ground pepper

Instructions:

Place the tofu, water and lemon juice in a blender or food processor and process until smooth. Place in a bowl and stir in remaining ingredients.

ORIENTAL SALAD DRESSING

Ingredients:

- 1/3 cup water
- 1 cup rice vinegar
- 1/4 cup low sodium soy sauce
- 1 teaspoon crushed red pepper (optional)
- 1 teaspoon crushed garlic
- 1 teaspoon crushed ginger root
- 1 teaspoon guar gum (a thickener)

Instructions:

Combine all ingredients in a small jar with a lid and shake until well mixed.

BALSAMIC VINAIGRETTE

Ingredients:

1 cup balsamic vinegar
1 cup cold water
1/2 cup Agave nectar or honey
1 teaspoon minced fresh ginger
1 teaspoon minced fresh garlic

Instructions:
Combine all ingredients in a blender jar and process until well blended. Chill before serving.

THAI CHILI DRESSING

Ingredients:

1 cup Mae Ploy Sweet Chili Sauce
1 cup water
1 tablespoon minced fresh ginger
Pinch of cilantro

Instructions:

Place all ingredients in a blender jar and process until blended.

SWEET POTATO HUMMUS

Perhaps this is more of a spread than a sauce but I have put this on potatoes and even rubbed it into a salad and it was great.

INGREDIENTS

1 1/4 cups mashed yam/sweet potato
2-3 cloves garlic
1 15 oz. can sodium free chickpeas/garbanzos, drained (reserve some liquid and set aside)
2-3 tbsp chickpea liquid
3 tsp apple cider vinegar
1 tablespoon tahini
1 teaspoon cumin
1/2 tsp curry powder
1/2 tsp smoked paprika
1/4-1/2 teaspoon Herbamare or salt (or to taste)
Fresh ground pepper to taste

Directions:

Poke holes in yam/sweet potato and bake at 400 F/205 C for about 45-60 minutes (till soft). Set aside when cool.

Pulse garlic in food processor until chopped and then add remaining ingredients.

Process until smooth and adjust consistency as desired with reserved chickpea liquid. Adjust seasonings to taste.

ASIAN STIR FRY IN TAHINI SAUCE

INGREDIENTS

- 1/3-1/2 cup water (only use higher amount for low powered blender)
- 2 tbsp tahini
- 2 large medjool dates, pitted, and chopped
- 1 large clove of garlic
- 2 tsp of fresh chopped ginger
- 1 1/2 tbsp low sodium tamari or soy sauce (gluten free if desired)

PREPARATIONS

Combine sauce ingredients in a Vita-Mix or blender and blend until smooth.

PIZZA SAUCE

INGREDIENTS

- 1 can of tomato paste
- 6 tbsp of water with 1/2 tsp Better Than Bouillon Vegetable base OR 6 tbsp water mixed with 1/2 cube bouillon
- 1 tbsp liquid sweetener (honey, agave, brown rice syrup)
- 3/4 tsp dried oregano
- 1/2 tsp freeze dried garlic or garlic powder
- 2 twists of ground black pepper
- dash of smoked paprika
- dash of salt (optional)
- sprinkle of chilli flakes (optional)

PREPARATION

1. Open the can of tomato paste and scoop into a bowl. Add all of the ingredients to the bowl and stir to combine. Taste test, adding additional seasonings if desired.

LOW FAT VEGAN CHEESE-ISH SAUCE

INGREDIENTS

- 1 cup almond milk, unsweetened original
- 1/4 cup nutritional yeast flakes
- 1/4 tsp smoked paprika
- 1/2 tsp miso paste
- Fresh ground pepper (optional)
- 1 1/2 tbsp whole wheat flour (optional)

PREPARATION

Add almond milk to a sauce pan and heat over medium heat until warm.
Sprinkle in the nutritional yeast and smoked paprika. Whisk it in.
Add the miso paste (break up).
Heat through a little and continue to whisk.
Taste test and add a little more smoked paprika and some ground pepper if desired.
Gently sprinkle in the flour and whisk in to combine.
Heat through for a minute or two until it's thickened. (Stir to prevent from sticking and burning)

BARBECUED BEAN SAUCE

Try this on baked potatoes. You will love it.

INGREDIENTS

- 1 onion, chopped
- 1 teaspoon minced fresh garlic
- ⅓ cup water
- 1 15 ounce can fire roasted chopped tomatoes with green chilies
- 1 teaspoon chili powder
- ¼ teaspoon chipotle chili powder
- ¼ teaspoon ground cumin
- 1 15 ounce can black beans, drained and rinsed
- 1 15 ounce can pinto beans, drained and rinsed
- 1 15 ounce can white beans, drained and rinsed
- 1 10 ounce package frozen mixed vegetables, thawed
- ½ cup vegetable broth
- ¼ cup barbecue sauce
- dash or two of hot sauce (optional)

PREPARATIONS

Place the onion, garlic and water in a large pot.
Cook, stirring occasionally for 5 minutes.
Add tomatoes and seasonings.
Mix well, then add the remaining ingredients.
Cook, stirring occasionally for 15 minutes.

BUTTER-LIKE SAUCE

INGREDIENTS

- ½ cup cashews
- 1 cup vegetable broth
- ½ cup water

Place the ingredients in a blender (high speed for about 7-10 minutes), food processor or Vitamix (highest speed possible for about 5 minutes)
Blend until completely smooth
Strain to remove any chunks of cashews

WARNING: This has a high fat content because of the cashews. You could add water or vegetable broth to cut down on the fat content but the sauce will be thinner.

AVOCADO SAUCE

INGREDIENTS

-
- 1 ripe avocado
- 3 tablespoons fresh cilantro
- 1/3 cup water
- ½ to ¾ teaspoon Tabasco sauce
- ½ teaspoon vinegar
- 1 teaspoon soy sauce

Peel and pit the avocado and place in a food processor.
Add the remaining ingredients and process until smooth.

GRAVY FOR MASHED POTATOES

INGREDIENTS

- ¼ cup whole wheat pastry flour
- 1 ½ cups vegetable broth
- ½ cup water
- 2 tablespoons tahini
- 3 tablespoons tamari or soy sauce
- freshly ground pepper to taste

PREPARATION

Place the flour in a non-stick frying pan.
Cook and stir over medium heat until the flour becomes a golden brown.
Slowly whisk in the vegetable broth and water.
After it is quite smooth, add the tahini and tamari or soy sauce.
Continue to whisk until mixture boils and is smooth and thick.
Season with freshly ground black pepper.

BOMBAY INDIAN VEGETABLE SAUCE

This looks more complicated than it is. Once you have made it one time you will make it over and over. Serve it on brown rice.

INGREDIENTS

- 1 teaspoon coriander seeds
- ½ teaspoon cumin seeds
- ½ teaspoon fennel seeds
- ½ teaspoon fenugreek seeds
- 6 whole green cardamoms
- ½ teaspoon turmeric
- ½ teaspoon freshly ground black pepper
- 3 tablespoons vegetable broth
- 1 large onion, cut in half lengthwise, then thinly sliced into crescents
- 3 cloves garlic, minced
- ½ cinnamon stick
- 1 red bell pepper, cut into ½ inch pieces
- 1 yellow bell pepper, cut into ½ inch pieces
- 2 jalapeno peppers, seeded and thinly sliced
- 3 large portobello mushrooms, cut in half, then thickly sliced
- 1 28 ounce can diced tomatoes, drained (reserve the juice)
- 1 15 ounce can garbanzo beans, drained and rinsed
- 4 cups fresh baby spinach (one 6 ounce bag)
- 2 tablespoons mango chutney
- 1/3 cup chopped fresh cilantro

PREPARATIONS

Place the 4 kinds of seeds and the cardamom into a dry non-stick frying pan.
Cook and stir for about 1 minute.
Remove from heat, cool, then crush using a mortar and pestle. Mix in the turmeric and black pepper.
Set aside.

Place the vegetable broth in a large pot.
Add the onion, garlic and cinnamon stick.
Cook, stirring frequently, for about 5 minutes.
Add the three kinds of peppers and the mushrooms.
Cook and stir for 3 more minutes.
Add the tomatoes, garbanzos, spinach, chutney, and ¼ cup of the reserved tomato juice.
Cook and stir for another 3-4 minutes.
Season with a bit more pepper and some salt (OPTIONAL)
Stir in the cilantro and let rest for a minute before serving.

QUICK VEGETABLE TOPPING

This is so easy there is no excuse to not give it a try.
Eat it just like this or on your baked potatoes or cooked whole grains.

INGREDIENTS

- 2 - 14.5 ounce cans chopped stewed tomatoes
- 1 - 15 ounce can cooked beans (black, white, pinto, garbanzo, any beans you like)

- 1 -10 ounce bag frozen corn kernels (or green peas, green beans, etc)

PREPARATION

Place all the ingredients in a medium saucepan
cook over medium heat for about 7 minutes until heated through.
Stir occasionally.

53. SNACKS

Your first and best choice for snacks is always fresh vegetables. Wash and prepare them to eat as soon as you bring them home from the market to make it easy for you later.

Dipping them in a no-fat hummus will make them more exciting.

Try the following:

- Sugar Snap Peas
- Carrot Sticks
- Celery Sticks
- Cucumber Slices
- Cherry Tomatoes
- Bell pepper slices
- Strawberries and berries
- Fresh sliced apples
- FROZEN GRAPES

OIL-FREE CHICKPEA HUMMUS

INGREDIENTS

- 1 15 oz./425 g can chickpeas (no salt) or 1 3/4 cup of fresh cooked chickpeas
- 1-2 small cloves of garlic (to taste)
- 1 1/2 tbsp filtered water
- 3-4 tbsp lemon juice (to taste)
- 1/4 tsp Herbamare (original) or Mrs. Dash Table Blend
- Fresh ground pepper (to taste)

PREPARATION

Drain and rinse the canned chickpeas
Add the garlic clove(s) to the food processor and pulse until chopped up.
Add the chickpeas, filtered water, lemon juice and pulse the chickpeas until they are fairly broken up.
Taste test and add more lemon if desired.
Add Herbamare (if desired) or Mrs. Dash Table Blend and a little fresh ground pepper.
Let it run until as smooth as you like it.

LEMON-OATMEAL COOKIES

INGREDIENTS

- 10 dates, pitted
- 1 cup unsweetened applesauce
- 1½ teaspoons apple cider vinegar
- 1 cup rolled oats
- 1 cup oat flour
- ½ cup quick-cooking oats
- ¾ cup roughly chopped walnuts (optional)
- 2 tablespoons grated lemon zest (2 lemons)
- 2 teaspoons natural cocoa powder
- 1 teaspoon vanilla powder
- ½ teaspoon baking soda
- Pinch of sea salt

PREPARATION

Preheat the oven to 275°F. Line 2 baking sheets with parchment paper.

Place the dates in a medium bowl and cover with hot water.
Set aside to soak for 20 minutes.
Drain any excess water from the bowl and transfer the dates to a blender or food processor.
Add the applesauce and vinegar and blend into a paste. Set aside.

In a large bowl, stir together the rolled oats, oat flour, quick-cooking oats, walnuts, lemon zest, cocoa powder, vanilla powder, baking soda, and salt.
Add the date and applesauce paste and use a wooden spoon to mix lightly but well. The mixture will be somewhat dry.

Make golf-ball-size portion of dough with your hands. Roll it into a ball and then pat it flat; (do this gently).
Place the round on the prepared baking sheet.

Bake until the tops of the cookies appear crispy and browned, 35 to 45 minutes.
Transfer to a wire rack to cool.

TERIYAKI VEGGIE CRUNCH ROLL

INGREDIENTS

RICE INGREDIENTS:
- 1 cup organic short grain brown rice
- 1½ tablespoons organic rice vinegar
- 1 tablespoon evaporated cane sugar
- ¼ teaspoon sea salt

FILLING INGREDIENTS:
- 1 small Japanese yam, roasted
- ½ ripe avocado
- 1 carrot, cut into thin strips
- ½ cucumber, peeled and cut into thin strips

- 3-4 toasted nori sheets
- ¾ cup organic crispy brown rice cereal

½ cup pickled ginger

TERIYAKI SAUCE INGREDIENTS:

- ½ cup wheat-free organic tamari
- ⅓ cup evaporated cane sugar
- 2 teaspoons brown rice vinegar
- 2 teaspoons pickled ginger, diced
- ¼ teaspoon garlic powder
- 2 tablespoons pineapple juice
- ½ teaspoon yuzu juice (optional)
- 2 teaspoons arrowroot powder, plus 1 tablespoons water, whisked

PREPARATION

Roast Japanese yam at 375°F for 45 minutes, or until soft. Peel and dice when cool and set aside in bowl.

In a medium saucepan, add 2 cups water and rice and cook according to directions.
When cooked, transfer rice into a large bowl.
With a wooden paddle, incorporate vinegar, sugar and sea salt into rice until slightly sticky, stirring vigorously. Let cool. Set aside.

For teriyaki sauce:

In small pot over medium heat add tamari, sugar, vinegar, ginger, garlic powder, pineapple juice and yuzu, if using. Whisk.
Cook for about 3 minutes, add arrowroot slurry and whisk.
Cook about 30 more seconds.

To roll sushi:
- Place sheet of toasted nori (shiny side down) on roller.
- With damp hands, spread cooked rice evenly over nori, leaving ½ inch on top portion of nori bare.
- Sprinkle with generous helping of crispy rice cereal.
- Flip sushi over onto plastic wrap lined sushi roller.
-
- Place small amount cooked yam, avocado, carrots and cucumber in a horizontal line, about 1 inch from base of nori.

- Turn sushi roller with fillings vertical to your body and slowly lift sides of sushi roller while making small rocking motions to align fillings.
- Using roller, tuck in filling until completely closed, allowing remaining top 3 inches of nori with rice to be exposed.
- Now fully enclose roll and squeeze gently.
- Slowly rock sushi using roller, until it forms a round shape.
- Gently press to seal, and round out sushi.

- Slide onto clean surface, and with a serrated damp knife, cut into 1 inch thick slices.

Drizzle with teriyaki sauce. Serve with ginger.

54. DESSERTS

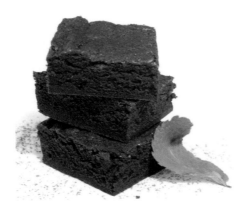

AMAZING BROWNIES

INGREDIENTS:

- 15 ounce can salt free Black Beans (rinsed and drained)
- 1.5 cups date paste (see recipe below)
- 3/4 cup unsweetened almond milk
- 2 tablespoons ground flax seeds
- 1 Tablespoon alcohol-free Vanilla Extract
- 1 teaspoon aluminum-free baking powder
- ½ teaspoon baking soda
- ½ cup cocoa or cacao powder
- ¾ gluten free oats, ground into a flour
- 1 cup non-dairy vegan chocolate chips* (optional)
- ½ cup finely chopped unsalted pistachios (optional)

PREPARATION

Preheat oven to 350.
Place beans and date paste and almond milk in a food processor fitted with the "S" blade and process until smooth.
Add the flax seeds, extracts, baking powder and soda and cocoa powder and process again.

Add ground oats and process very briefly, just until combined. Pour batter into an 9 x 9 square silicone baking pan.

Sprinkle with nuts and or chocolate chips, if using and gently press the toppings down with the palm of your hand.

Bake for 30-35 minutes until middle does not jiggle and toothpick inserted comes out clean.

Cool before cutting.

WARNING ABOUT CHOCOLATE CHIPS: Sunspire brand is are made with barley malt which means it contains gluten. All of the gluten-free chocolate chips contain sugar as the first ingredients

DATE PASTE

Great way to sweeten desserts without using sugar. You might want to make a big batch of this so you have it on hand when you need it.

INGREDIENTS:

- One pound of pitted dates
- One cup of liquid (water, unsweetened non-dairy milk, unsweetened juice)

PREPARATION

Soak dates in liquid overnight or for several hours until much of the liquid is absorbed. In food processor fitted with the "S" blade, process dates and liquid until completely smooth.

Store in the refrigerator.

TRIPLE APPLE CAKE

INGREDIENTS:

- 3 Apples, thinly sliced (about 4 cups)
- 2 ounces of dried apple rings, approximately 1 cup, packed and snipped into small pieces
- 1 and 1/2 cup of applesauce
- 6 Tablespoons ground flax seed
- 1 teaspoon sodium free baking powder
- 1 teaspoon sodium free baking soda
- 1 Tablespoon Alcohol-free vanilla
- 1 Tablespoon Apple Pie spice (or 2.5 teaspoons of cinnamon plus 1/2 teaspoon nutmeg)
- 2 cups gluten free oats

PREPARATION

Preheat oven to 350.
Mix all ingredients together and pour in a 9 inch square silicone baking dish.
Bake for 30-35 minutes.

Let cool before slicing (chill for the best texture).

HEALTHY PUMPKIN PIE DAIRY-FREE ICE CREAM

INGREDIENTS:

1/4 cup orange juice
1/4 cup vanilla almond milk, unsweetened
8 ounces of carrots (approximately 1.5 cups), frozen
1 teaspoon roasted cinnamon
2-3 large ripe bananas, frozen (peel before freezing)

PREPARATION

Mix all ingredients except for the bananas in a high powered blender and blend until smooth.
Add 2-3 large, frozen bananas and blend until creamy.

APPLE PIE ICE CREAM

INGREDIENTS

1 Large Sweet Apple, sliced and frozen (at least 10 ounces)
2 Large Ripe Bananas, peeled and frozen
1 cup unsweetened almond milk
2 teaspoons alcohol-free vanilla
1 teaspoon apple pie spice or cinnamon
½ cup apple juice
½ cup nondairy milk

PREPARATION

In a high powered blender blend the apple, nondairy milk and spices until smooth.
Add the frozen bananas and blend until thick and creamy.

CREAMY BLUEBERRY PARFAIT

INGREDIENTS: Pudding

3.4 cup millet
3.5 cups unsweetened nondairy milk
6 Tablespoons date paste (see recipe above)
1 Tablespoon alcohol free vanilla
1 teaspoon roasted cinnamon
½ teaspoon ground cardamom
PREPARATION

In a blender, blend nondairy milk, date paste, vanilla and spices until full.

In a medium saucepan, bring millet and the contents of the blender to a full boil.

Reduce heat and simmer for 25-30 minutes until thick.
Remove from heat.

FRUIT TOPPINGS INGREDIENTS:

2 cups unsweetened pomegranate juice
2 Tablespoons date paste (see recipe above)
4 Tablespoons cornstarch dissolved in 4 Tablespoons water
1 cup blueberries

PREPARATION:
In a medium saucepan dissolve date paste into the pomegranate juice and reduce until you have ½ a cup. Slowly stir in cornstarch until mixture thickens, then gently stir in blueberries.
Remove from heat.

ASSEMBLY:
Distribute pudding mixture evenly into 4-6 glasses.
Evenly distribute the fruit topping on each of the parfaits.
Chill before serving

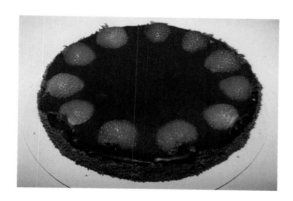

STRAWBERRY CHOCOLATE CHEESECAKE

Okay, folks. I paid $20 for this recipe. I had to spend the money to learn the secret!!!! Here it is.

INGREDIENTS – Crust

2 cups of almond flour
12 ounces of pitted dates (about 2 cups tightly packed)
1 Tablespoon alcohol free vanilla

PREPARATION:

In a food processor fitted with the "S" blade process the dates and almond flour until a ball forms.
Add the vanilla and briefly process again.
Evenly press into an 8 or 9 inch Springform pan lined with parchment paper.

INGREDIENTS – Filling

8 ounces of nondairy cream cheese
12.3 ounces package of Extra Firm Silken Tofu
½ cup of cocoa powder
¾ cup of date syrup (Whole Foods carries this or get online)
10 ounces of nondairy grain sweetened Sunspire chocolate chips
1 Tablespoon Alcohol free vanilla

PREPARATION:

Over a double boiler or very carefully in a nonstick pan, mix the chocolate chips and date syrup and melt over low heat until smooth.

Place in a food processor fitted with the "S" blade with the remaining filling ingredients and process until smooth.

Pour evenly over crust and top with strawberries.
Drizzle with the melted chocolate topping.

INGFREDIENTS – Topping

2 pounds strawberries (medium to large, preferred)
2 ounces of a 100% cacao chocolate bar
¼ cup date syrup
¼ cup nondairy milk

PREPARATION

Cut the stems off of the strawberries so the top of the strawberries will lay flat on the cake.

Place all of the strawberries on top of the cake, pushing into the filling slightly.
Over a double boiler or very carefully in a nonstick pan, melt chocolate, plant milk and date syrup.

Mix until smooth.

Drizzle the melted chocolate over the cake.

Refrigerate until firm, about 4 hours.

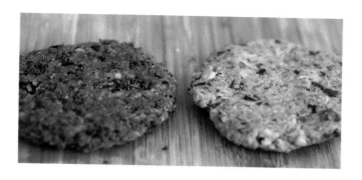

55. "Meat" Loaf Cakes

INGREDIENTS

¼ c uncooked quinoa + ½ c water
2 15-oz cans unsalted kidney beans, rinsed and drained½ c finely diced raw onion
1 c finely diced raw button mushrooms
1 tsp salt free seasoning
6 Tbsp corn or whole wheat flour
1 batch of sweet sauce for "meat" loaves (see recipe below)

PREPARATION

Preheat oven to 425 F.

Rinse quinoa, drain well, and combine with water in a small saucepan.
Cover and bring to a boil, then reduce heat and simmer 20 minutes, until liquid is absorbed and quinoa is tender. Remove from heat.

While quinoa is cooking:
In a small skillet add about one tablespoon of water or vegetable broth and saute diced onions and mushrooms for 6-7 minutes, until both are tender and onions begin to brown (add a little more water if they stick too much).
Remove from heat.

In a large bowl, mash kidney beans with a fork until most of the beans have broken open.

Add 6 Tbsp corn flour, and 3 Tbsp sweet sauce (recipe below) to the mashed beans. Stir to combine, do not over-smash the beans (The consistency will look a little dry).

Add cooked quinoa, mushrooms, and onions, and mix gently, with your hands.

Line 8 cups in a muffin tin with 2-inch-wide strips of parchment paper arranged in X's.

Press bean mixture firmly into the lined cups, until almost flush with the rim of each cup. Should fill 8 cups.

Bake 5 minutes, then carefully remove each cake from the muffin tin and invert onto a parchment-lined baking sheet.

Spread approx. 1 Tbsp of sweet sauce over the top of each cake.

Bake cakes for another 15-17 minutes, until sides of cakes are lightly browned.

Sweet Sauce for "Meat" Loaves

INGREDIENTS

10 dried dates, chopped
½ c ketchup
2 tsp ground dried mustard
½ tsp allspice
½ tsp ground cloves

PREPARATION

Using a mini food processor combine sauce ingredients until smooth.

Serves: 4 (makes 8 mini-cakes)

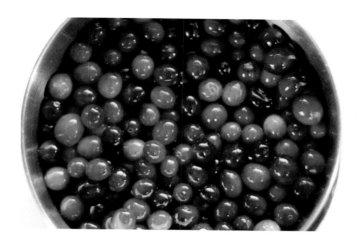

56. Raw Cranberry Relish

1 orange, peeled

1 cup fresh or frozen cranberries

1 medium apple, quartered

5 pitted dates (or to taste)

1/3 cup pecans or walnuts (optional)

Zest of 1 orange

Place all ingredients in a food processor and pulse till you feel it looks done.

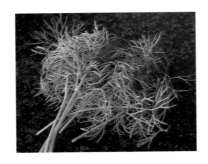

57. Potato and Grilled Corn Salad with Fresh Dill

INGREDIENTS

4 cobs of corn, husked
2 pounds small white potatoes, washed
3 green onions, sliced
2 tablespoons dijon mustard
1/4 teaspoon salt
1/4 teaspoon freshly ground black pepper
1/4 cup white wine vinegar
2 tablespoons chopped fresh dill

PREPARATION

Place corn on grill over medium-high heat. Grill until tender and slightly charred, about 10 minutes.
Remove from heat, let cool slightly.
Cut off kernels.
Place into a large bowl.

Boil potatoes until tender, about 15 minutes.
Drain and slice in half.

Add to the bowl of corn, along with green onions, mustard, salt, pepper, vinegar and dill.

Toss all to combine well.

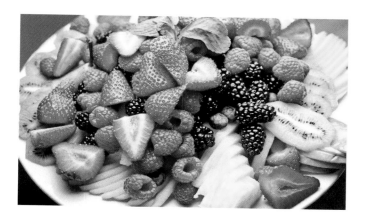

58. Fruit Salad On Wonderful Greens

INGREDIENTS:

2 c. loosely packed baby spinach
1/4 c. sprouts
1/4 c. cucumber, cut into 1 inch pieces
1 fresh peach, cut in 1 inch pieces
1/4 c. blueberries
1/4 c. fresh cut pineapple, cut in 1 inch pieces
1 T. pecan pieces (optional)
1 t. pumpkin seeds (optional)
juice from the freshly cut fruit (optional)

PREPARATION

Place spinach on plate. Top with cucumber and sprouts. Then add peach, blueberries and pineapple. Sprinkle with nuts and seeds. The fruit is the dressing so need to add more.

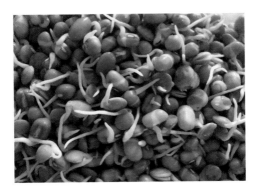

59. Cucumber and Mung Bean Sprout Salad

INGREDIENTS

2-3 large cucumbers
2 cups mung bean sprouts
3-4 cups fresh pea greens
4-5 fresh or canned water chestnuts
2 Tbs. light soy sauce (or wheat-free tamari)
1 Tbs. cider vinegar
1 Tbs. freshly minced garlic
several splashes to 1 tsp. Tabasco sauce
1 Tbs. black bean sauce
1/4 tsp. fresh ground pepper, optional

PREPARATION

Peel the cucumber, slice it down the middle and remove the seeds. Cut each half down the middle and slice these strips into bite sized pieces.

Toss cucumbers and mung bean sprouts into a large sealable container. Mix the dressing separately and pour over the veggies. Put the lid on the container and shake it. Put it in the fridge for 3 hours or over night.

Just before serving add the pea greens and peeled, chopped water chestnuts and shake the whole thing together again.

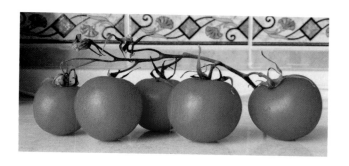

60. Tomato and Onion Salad with Tahini Dressing

INGREDIENTS

1 medium red or white onion, peeled and diced
[salt] and pepper to taste
1/2 garlic clove, peeled and minced, or to taste
1/3 cup tahini paste
1/2 teaspoon ground cumin
2 tablespoons fresh lemon juice, or more to taste
4 medium tomatoes, cored and chopped
1/2 cup fresh parsley leaves, chopped

PREPARATIONS

Soak onion in salted cold water while preparing other ingredients, about 30 minutes.

Whisk or blend together garlic, tahini and cumin, and add lemon juice; the mixture will become very thick. Thin with hot water, a tablespoon at a time, so the mixture can be spooned.

Season to taste with [salt] and pepper.

Toss onion, tomatoes and parsley with dressing.
Taste, adjust the seasonings and serve.

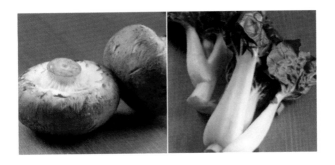

61. Kung Pao Vegetables

INGREDIENTS

- 8 oz Sliced Mushrooms
- 3/4 c Diced Carrots
- 3/4 c Diced Celery
- 3/4 c Diced Onion
- 8 oz Diced Water Chestnuts – see note
- 1/2 c Dry Roasted Peanuts (optional) – see note
- 3 Cloves Garlic Minced
- 3 Leaves/Stalks Bok Choy Diced

-
- 3T Rice Wine or Sake
- 3T Low Sodium Soy Sauce or Tamari
- 2T Rice Vineagar
- 2T Cornstarch in 1/4 c Water
- Sriracha or Sambal Oelek to taste

PREPARATION

Place the sliced Mushrooms in a dry wok or pan and stir until the Mushrooms release their liquid.
Add the Carrots, Celery, and Onions and cook until the colors brighten.
Add the Water Chestnuts, Peanuts, Garlic and Bok Choy stalks and cook until heated through.
Add the Bok Choy leaves and cook until slightly wilted.

Mix together the Rice Wine, Soy Sauce and Rice Vinegar.
Pour over the vegetables and stir cook until slightly bubbly.
Add the cornstarch dissolved in water to thicken the sauce.
Add Asian Chile Paste to taste.

Serve over Brown Rice

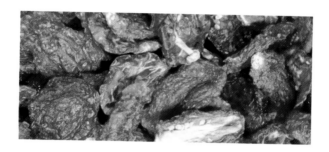

62. Mushroom Sun-dried Tomato Oat Risotto

INGREDIENTS

1 to 2 tablespoons water or veggie broth
½ small onion, minced
2 cloves of garlic, minced
1 cup minced mushrooms
¼ cup minced green bell pepper
1 teaspoon dried basil
1 teaspoon dried oregano
½ teaspoon dried marjoram
⅛ teaspoon ground rosemary or 1/4 teaspoon regular rosemary
1 cup Steel-cut Oats
2 tablespoons minced sun-dried tomatoes
4 to 5 cups water (as needed – see instructions)
2 tablespoons nutritional yeast
(salt) and pepper, to taste

PREPARATION

Water saute the onions over medium heat, cook until translucent then add the garlic, mushrooms, bell pepper and herbs. Saute for 5 to 20 minutes, until the mushrooms have browned and released their juices.

Add in the oats and stir to prevent them from burning. Cook until lightly toasted, about 3 minutes.

Add the sun dried tomatoes and 1 cup of water. Simmer over medium heat stirring often to keep the mixture from burning on the bottom.

Once the first cup of water has been absorbed by the oats add a second cup of water and keep stirring. Add the third cup of water once the second is absorbed and keep stirring.

Once the third cup is absorbed add one more cup water and after it's absorbed try a piece of the oats to see if it's cooked through.
(chewy texture and not mushy).

Right before serving add the nutritional yeast, salt and pepper.

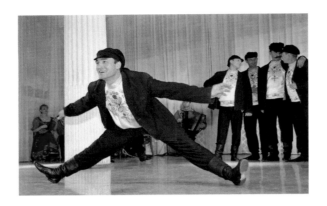

63. Russian Piaf

INGREDIENT

- 2 c short-grain brown rice
- 2 Tbsp sliced almonds
- 1 large onion (diced)
- 4 medium carrots (grated)
- 2 cloves of garlic
- 3 Tbsp golden raisins
- 1 tsp Cumin
- No-Salt seasoning & pepper
- water or veggie stock

PREPARATION

Cook rice and almonds separately (according to the directions on rice).
In a covered, deep and nonstick pan, add a little water or vegetable broth and get it hot. Saute the onion and garlic.

After 4 min, add the carrots and cook covered for 10 min, stirring often.
Then add the raisins and cumin. Mix and cook covered for 5 more min.

Add the cooked rice and almonds, and about add 3/4 c hot water. The amount of water you add depends somewhat on how much liquid was included with the rice.

Now mix and cook covered for 15 min at low-to-medium heat.
Remove from heat and no-salt seasoning & pepper to taste. Should be sweet (from the raisins)more so than salty, but you can adjust the seasonings to suite your taste.

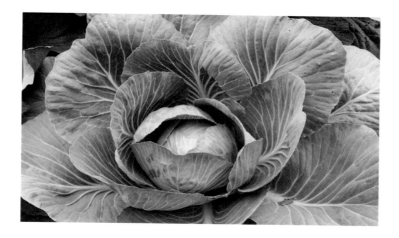

64. Green Cabbage Soup

INGREDIENTS

- 10 cups water
- 3 cups vegetable stock
- 1 green cabbage, chopped fine
- 5 celery stalks chopped fine
- 4 medium carrots diced
- 4 Spanish onions diced
- 2 cups greens (spinach, kale, cress, collard greens, etc.)
-
- 1 1/2 tsp. no-salt seasoning
- 3/4 -1 tsp. fresh ground black pepper
- 3 T. fresh sage, chopped
- 2 t. dried marjoram
- 2 tsp. crushed dried rosemary or 1 T. chopped fresh

PREPARATION

Let all of the ingredients simmer for about 3 hours, adding
1 1/2 cups of red, wild, brown rice about 1 hour into the simmering.
Soup should have been cooking at least 4 hours.

Near serving time, stir in 12-24 ounces plain [non-dairy] yogurt.
2 T. white wine or wine vinegar

Garnish with 5-6 minced green/spring onions, about a 1/3 cup each bowl of soup.

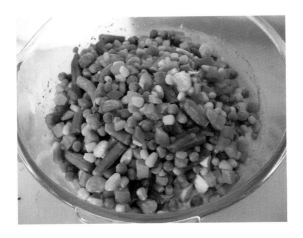

65. Vegetable Pot Pie

INGREDIENTS

- Topping
- 1 Tbsp ground flax seed
- 3 Tbsp water
- ½ c corn meal
- ¼ c brown rice flour
- ¼ c amaranth flour
- 1½ tsp baking powder
- ¼ c apple sauce
- ½ c unsweetened nondairy milk

Filling
- 5 c frozen mixed vegetables + ¼ c water
- 1½ c frozen mixed mushrooms OR washed and sliced fresh button mushrooms
- 1 Tbsp nutritional yeast
- ½ tsp onion powder
- ½ tsp garlic powder
- ⅛ tsp ground pepper
- 2 Tbsp corn starch + 2 Tbsp cold water
- Cooking liquid from frozen vegetables
- ¾ c unsweetened nondairy milk

PREPARATION

Preheat oven to 400F

In a small microwaveable bowl, mix together 1 Tbsp ground flax seed and 3 Tbsp water. Microwave for 30-45 seconds, or until gooey paste. Set aside.

Place the frozen vegetables and mushrooms (fresh or frozen) in a microwaveable, deep-dish pie pan. Add ¼ c water, invert a dinner plate over the top, and microwave on high for 10 minutes, stirring after 5 minutes. Reserve the cooking liquid.

Topping
Prepare dry ingredients: In a large bowl, whisk together the corn meal, brown rice flour, amaranth flour, baking powder.

In a separate small bowl, add the apple sauce, ½ c nondairy milk and flax seed paste. Mix well with a fork.

Sauce
Once veggies are done cooking, carefully drain the cooking liquid into a measuring cup. Add nondairy milk to the cooking liquid until you have 1 c liquid total. Pour into a small pot. Add nutritional yeast, onion powder, garlic powder, salt, and black pepper to the pot, and whisk to combine.

Bring to a boil.

Measure 2 Tbsp of cornstarch and 2 Tbsp cold water into the measuring cup and mix thoroughly with a fork. Whisking constantly, add the cornstarch slurry to the boiling liquid.
Remove from heat after 5-10 seconds.

Put it all together
Add thickened sauce to vegetables in pie dish and stir gently to combine.

Pour the wet topping ingredients into the dry topping ingredients and stir until just combined.

Pour batter over top of vegetables in pie dish and smooth to the edges with a spatula.

Bake at 400F for 30-35 minutes, or until a toothpick inserted in the cornbread comes out clean.

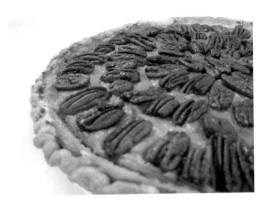

66. Sweet Potato-Pecan Pie

INGREDIENTS

- 1½ cups (packed) cooked sweet potato or yam (about 1 pound uncooked)
- 4 ounces dates (about 8 Medjool or 16 Deglet Noor), pitted and quartered
- ¾ cup nondairy milk
- 1 teaspoon vanilla extract
- ¼ to ½ cup rolled oats, ground into flour (½ cup will result in a firmer filling)
- 1¼ teaspoon cinnamon
- ¼ teaspoon ground ginger
- ⅛ teaspoon ground clove
- ¼ cup pecan halves, chopped, plus 15 to 20 pecan halves to decorate the outside edge.

PREPARTION

Preheat oven to 375°F.

To bake the sweet potato or yam, place it onto a baking sheet and bake for 60 to 70 minutes, or until very soft when pierced with a knife.

Place the dates, nondairy milk, and vanilla extract into a blender (making sure to grind your oats first), and set aside for at least 15 minutes.
In a medium bowl, add the oat flour, cinnamon, ginger, and clove, and mix thoroughly with a fork.

Blend the dates, nondairy milk, and vanilla in a blender on high speed until smooth. Blend in the dry ingredients followed by the baked sweet potato or yam until the filling is very smooth.

Scrape into a pre-baked pie crust and smooth out evenly.

Arrange the pecan halves around the outside and the chopped pecans in the middle.

Gently wrap a few strips of foil around the top edge of the pie so the crust does not get overcooked.

Bake for 25 to 30 minutes. Remove from the oven and remove the foil strips, and let cool before slicing.

Steps 2: Place the dough on a piece of parchment paper.

Step 3: Place a piece of parchment paper on top of the dough, and roll it out into a circle using a rolling pin, to about 1/8-inch thick.

Step 4: Use the pie pan as a guide in cutting the crust.

Step 5: Flip the pie pan, the crust and the parchment paper and peel away the top parchment paper using a spatula on the underside to loosen the crust from the mat.

Step 6: The crust should now be laying on top of the pie pan.

Step 7: Gently ease the crust into the contours of the pie pan.

Step 8: Trim off any extra, overhanging crust, being careful not to secure the crust under the pan lip.

Step 9: Cover the uncooked crust with foil and loosely curl the edges under. Bake for 10 minutes.

Step 10: After the crust has baked and cooled for at least 10 minutes, spread the filling evenly inside the crust.

Step 11: Top with pecans.

Step 12: Place a few aluminum foil strips around the edges to keep the crust from over-browning.

Step 13: Bake for 30 minutes.

Cut the pie after it has cooled.

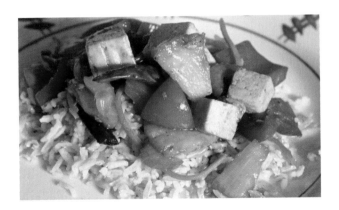

67. Pineapple Stir-Fry

INGREDIENTS

- 1 cup chopped yellow onion
- 1 tablespoon minced garlic
- 2 medium carrots, thinly sliced
- 2 ribs celery, sliced
- 1 medium red bell pepper, seeded and chopped
- 6 medium white mushrooms, sliced
- 1 cup fresh pineapple juice (or unsweetened juice from one 20-ounce can)
- 2 cups cubed fresh pineapple (or one 20-ounce can)
- 1 teaspoon freshly minced ginger
- 2 teaspoons brown rice vinegar
- ¼-½ teaspoon red pepper flakes
- 4 green onions, chopped
- 4 cups cooked brown rice or noodles to serve 4

INSTRUCTIONS

Chop and prepare all ingredients before starting, as this dish cooks up quickly.

Place 1 tablespoon of water into a large skillet on high heat. When the water begins to sputter, add the onion and cook stirring for 1 to 2 minutes.
Add the garlic, carrot, celery, bell pepper, and mushrooms, and cook stirring for 2 to 3 minutes.

Add a little of the pineapple juice gradually as needed to keep the vegetables from sticking.

Add the pineapple, ginger, vinegar, red pepper flakes, and any remaining pineapple juice, and cook stirring for another 2 minutes. Stir in the green onion last, just before serving.

Serve immediately over hot, cooked brown rice or noodles.

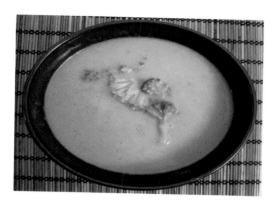

68. Broccoli Soup

INGREDIENTS

- 6 cups water
- 1½ pounds Yukon gold potatoes (2 to 3 large), cut into chunks (skin on)
- 1 medium yellow onion, chopped
- 2 teaspoons ground coriander
- 2 teaspoons granulated garlic
- 1 teaspoon granulated onion
- 1 teaspoon no-salt poultry seasoning
- 1½ pounds broccoli (1 to 2 heads), coarsely chopped
- 3 large Swiss chard leaves, ends trimmed and coarsely chopped

INSTRUCTIONS

In a large soup pot, add the water, potatoes, onion, coriander, granulated garlic and onion, and poultry seasoning, and bring to a boil.

Reduce heat to medium, and add the broccoli.

Cook covered for about 10 minutes, until the potatoes and broccoli are tender (stirring occasionally).

Stir in the chard and cook for an additional 5 minutes.

Remove from the heat and let stand for about 5 minutes.
Using an immersion blender, blend the soup right in the pot until smooth but still with some small lumps and chunks or a blender.

Serve immediately as is or topped with sliced or chopped tomatoes.

Serves: 6 to 8

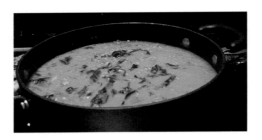

69. Tomato Rice Soup

INGREDIENTS

- 1 medium yellow or white onion, chopped (2 cups)
- 6½ cups water
- 1 can (15 ounces) Navy or white beans, drained and rinsed (or 1½ cups)
- ¾ cup uncooked, long-grain brown rice
- 2 cans (14.5 ounces each) unsalted diced tomatoes
- 2 ribs celery, chopped
- 5 medium white mushrooms, sliced (about 2 cups)
- 1 tablespoon dried Italian herb blend (dried oregano, basil, thyme, rosemary, sage, and/or parsley)
- 1½ teaspoons granulated garlic
- 4 leaves Swiss chard (or beet greens, collard greens, and kale), coarsely chopped (2 to 3 cups)
- 15 large leaves fresh basil, chopped (about 1 cup)

INSTRUCTIONS

Place 1 tablespoon of water into a soup pot on high heat. When the water begins to sputter, add the onion and cook stirring for 3 to 5 minutes, until the onions become softened.

Add the water, beans, rice, diced tomatoes (including juice), celery, mushrooms, dried Italian herbs, and granulated garlic, and stir. Bring to a boil, and then reduce heat to a simmer.

Cover and cook for 25 minutes.

Stir in the greens and cook covered for 10 more minutes. Stir in the basil and serve.

Serves: 6 to 8 (makes about 10 cups)

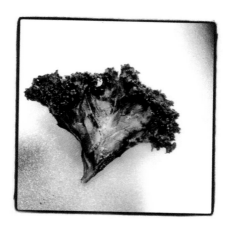

70. Baked Kale Chips

INGREDIENTS

*
* Fresh kale leaves
* Seasonings as desired
* Bragg Liquid Aminos or balsamic vinegar

Preheat oven to 225 degrees

Wash the kale well and leave some of the water clinging to the leaves. Strip the leaves from the thick stems and cut into uniform sized pieces.

Place on a non-stick baking sheet or on top of parchment paper on a regular baking sheet and sprinkle with seasonings of your choice.

Spray them with a light coating and a light dusting of seasoning.

Bake for about 30 minutes until crispy.

Store in a tightly covered container to keep them crispy.

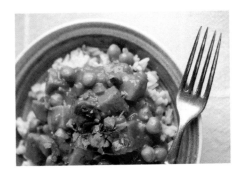

71. Chickpea and Sweet Potato Satay

INGREDIENTS

- 1/2 cup water
- 1 medium brown onion, sliced
- 1 clove garlic, peeled and crushed
- 1 tbsp. grated fresh ginger
- 1/4 tsp. red pepper flakes
- 1.5 pounds of sweet potatoes, peeled and cut into inch-thick pieces
- 1 red bell pepper, sliced
- 3 celery stalks, sliced
- 1 15 ounce can of chickpeas, drained and rinsed
- 2 tbsp. chopped fresh cilantro

For the Satay Sauce:
- 1 ½ tbsp. crunchy peanut butter
- 1 tbsp. salt-reduced soy sauce
- 2 tsp. rice vinegar or tamarind paste
- 2 tbsp. sweet chili sauce
- 1/4 tsp. ground coriander
- 4 tbsp. water

PREPARATION

Combine all ingredients for the satay sauce in a bowl and whisk to combine. Set aside.

Heat a large fry-pan or wok, add the 1/2 cup of water, onion, garlic, ginger and red pepper flakes; cook, stirring, for 3-4 minutes.

Add the sweet potato and cook for a further 12 minutes, adding more water as necessary to prevent sticking.

Add the bell pepper and celery and cook for 3-4 minutes, until slightly softened.

Add the chickpeas and satay sauce, and cook at a high heat for about a minute, until the sauce thickens.

Remove from the heat and serve immediately, sprinkled with fresh coriander.

Serves: 2

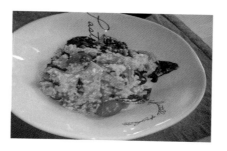

72. Millet and Black Bean Salad

INGREDIENTS

-
- 1 ½ cups cooked millet
- 1 15 ounce (425g) can black beans, drained and rinsed
- 2/3 cup corn kernels (fresh, canned or thawed frozen kernels)
- 2 small tomatoes, diced
- 1 medium carrot, grated
- ¼ tsp. dried garlic
- ¼ tsp. cayenne pepper
- 1 tsp. agave
- 3 tbsp. lemon juice
- 2 tbsp. chopped fresh coriander (cilantro)
- 1 tbsp. chopped jalapenos (optional)

PREPRATION

Combine all ingredients in a large bowl and mix until well combined.

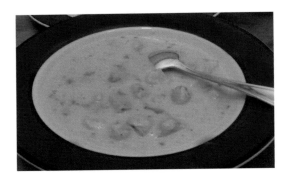

73. Potato Soup

INGREDIENTS

- 3 Lb. organic red potatoes, peeled and sliced
- 2 organic yellow corn ears
- 2 scallions
- 1 Tbsp. organic white onion, chopped
- 3 garlic cloves, chopped
- 1 cup organic carrots, finely chopped
- 4 cups, low sodium, organic vegetable broth
- 4 cups water
- 1 sprig cilantro
- ½ cup dehydrated or fresh Gallant Soldier herbs (guascas) (BUY ON AMAZON or use your favorite no salt seasoning)
- Capers to taste (optional)

PREPARATION

In a large pot, place water, vegetable broth, onion, carrot and cilantro to boil.
Meanwhile, place gallant soldier herbs in a bowl of warm water for about an hour.

Slice corn ears onto 4 pieces each. Add corn and sliced potatoes. Let soup simmer covered in medium heat for 90 minutes until soup thickens, stirring frequently.

Add gallant soldier and simmer for another 10 minutes in low heat. Top with capers.

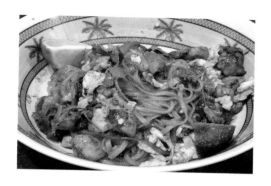

74. Pad Thai

INGREDIENTS

- ¼ lb thick rice noodles
- 2 tbsp low-sodium soy sauce
- 1 tbsp smooth peanut butter
- 1 tbsp sweet red chili sauce
- ¼ tsp granulated garlic powder
- ¼ tsp ground ginger
- ¼ tsp hot sauce
- 1 15-oz package of frozen vegetables
- 3 oz bean sprouts
- chopped raw peanuts
- lime wedge

Prepare rice noodles according to package directions.

In a small bowl, whisk 2 tbsp warm water, soy sauce, peanut butter, chili sauce, garlic powder, ginger, and hot sauce together until combined. It may appear too runny at first, but it's not. Taste, adding more hot sauce if desired.

Cook one 15-oz package of frozen stir-fry veggies according to package instructions.

Using tongs, add vegetables and toss prepared noodles with the sauce until all noodles are evenly coated.

Top with bean sprouts.
Garnish with chopped raw peanuts and a lime wedge.

Serves 2

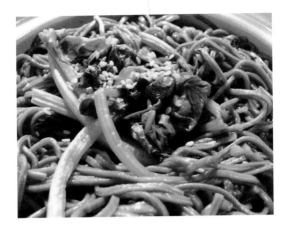

75. Noodles and Greens with Creamy Japanese Dressing

INGREDIENTS

- 8-9 ounces of uncooked soba noodles
- Add 1 large bunch of chopped hearty greens, such as kale or collards

Bring a large pot of water to a boil. Add uncooked soba noodles to the pot. Return to a boil and cook for about 5 minutes. Add chopped hearty greens.
Continue to cook, uncovered, stirring frequently to keep the greens under the water, for about 5 more minutes.

Drain and place in a bowl.

Creamy Japanese Dressing

INGREDIENTS

- ¼ cup soy sauce
- ¼ cup rice vinegar
- ¼ cup agave nectar
- 2 tablespoons tahini
- ½ cup silken tofu (optional)

Process in a high speed blender until smooth and creamy.

Toasted sesame process in a high speed blender, then add the remaining ingredients and process again until smooth.

76. Conclusion

I hope you have enjoyed these recipes. This is only a starting point into your new lifestyle round food. Now that you have some basic recipes, you can explore ways to change them to suit you.

Insulin resistance, diabetes and PCOS are difficult condition to live with, but what you eat will change everything about your quality of life. You will be able to lose the extra weight and maintain it now that you know what you should be eating. You don't have to become a diabetic and a woman with PCOS's can regulate her menstrual cycle.

I hope you explore the Resource Chapter to find the hard core research and explanations on why this way of eating is so helpful. Understanding the information can support you in your change.

If you are having trouble getting pregnant or would like to take a Chinese herbal formula for your health care needs send me an email at: patricia@fertilityformulas.com

♥

77. Helpful Resources

Nutrition Research review http://nutritionfacts.org/

Dr. Esselstyn Cartiologist http://www.dresselstyn.com/

Pamela Popper doctor of nutrition http://drpampopper.com/

Dr. McDougall Health and Medical Center https://www.drmcdougall.com

Doug Lisle, Ph.D. (Psychologist) http://www.healthpromoting.com

Forks Over Knives (documentary Film) http://www.forksoverknives.com/

Dr. Neal Barnard, Physicians Committee for Responible Medicine http://www.pcrm.org/

Whole food plant based chef AJ http://chefajwebsite.com/

Low Fat Chef http://lowfatveganchef.com/

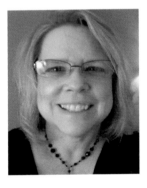

Contact me, Patricia Karnowski MSOM, LAc for custom made Chinese herbal formulas to help you get pregnant.
patricia@PCOSworld.com
patricia@fertilityformulas.com

♥

Go to pcosworld.com to view the videos by prominent doctors and researchers to get a better understanding of why a whole food plant based diet with no salt, oil or sugar is best for you.

♥